POCKET GUIDE TO
NATUROPATHIC MEDICINE

JUDITH BOICE, N.D.

The Crossing Press
Freedom, California

Cautionary note: The information contained within this book is in no way intended as a substitute for medical counseling. Please do not attempt self-treatment of a medical problem without consulting a qualified health practitioner.

For information on bulk purchases or group discounts for this and other Crossing Press titles, please contact our Special Sales Manager at 800-777-1048.

ISBN 0-89594-821-4

For my professors at the National College of Naturopathic Medicine, who have passed on the tradition of naturopathic medicine with the utmost dedication and integrity.

For my parents, who have been unfailingly supportive through my years of education.

For those who are searching for natural, non-invasive ways to support their health and well-being.

Acknowledgments

Giovanni Maciocia, *The Foundations of Chinese Medicine*. New York: Churchill, Livingstone, 1989, p. 312 (quoted on pp. 4–5).

Dr. Jared Zeff, for the "Paradigm of Health and Disease." I am indebted to you for your careful research and thoughtful reflection on the philosophy of naturopathic medicine, which led to the creation of this paradigm. You are an ongoing source of inspiration for me.

My thanks to Dr. James Sensenig for his careful review of the manuscript, and for his tireless dedication to the naturopathic profession.

My appreciation to Linda Gunnarson and the staff at The Crossing Press for their support in preparing this manuscript.

CONTENTS

Chapter One
Introduction to Naturopathic Medicine

Naturopathic medicine relies for its healing knowledge on the vast repository of wisdom innate in the Earth. When you begin working with naturopathic medicine, you will be using the oldest, most clinically researched medicine available—natural therapeutics that have been applied effectively for tens of thousands of years—combined with the best of contemporary research and technology.

Naturopathic medicine is a system of classical medicine defined by its philosophy. The term "classical" more fully captures the essence of naturopathic medicine than do the terms "alternative" or "complementary." The roots of naturopathic medicine reach back to classical times, when physicians studied the processes of health as well as the processes of disease. Those roots extend even deeper into the soil of time, to an era when humans understood the healing power in their own bodies, as well as in the plants and elements that surround them. This innate healing power, or natural intelligence, directs the body to regenerate and rebalance.

Many techniques or healing modalities fit under the umbrella of naturopathic medicine. The philosophy of naturopathic medicine provides the link that unifies this group of diverse practices. A core aspect of this philosophy, outlined more fully below, is that treatment must be individualized to meet the needs of a particular patient. Naturopathic medicine treats diseases by treating people.

Ten people with similar cold or flu symptoms may walk into my office, and those ten patients probably will walk out with ten different treatment plans, each tailored to suit a particular set of needs.

This diversity in treatment methods makes naturopathic medicine difficult for some people to understand. Legislative bodies understand other healing modalities—acupuncture, for example—more readily because the method of healing is consistent from patient to patient. Acupuncturists use needles. Chiropractic physicians administer "force" or "non-force" methods of adjustment. Medical doctors prescribe pharmaceutical drugs and surgery.

A naturopathic physician, however, has a vast array of potential treatments from which to choose. Naturopathic medical students study all of the medical sciences, including clinical and physical diagnosis, pathology, anatomy (with dissection lab), biochemistry, physiology, pharmacology, and specialty areas such as pediatrics, gynecology, and cardiology—in short, all of the courses taught at any medical school. In addition, we spend several hundred hours studying courses that have disappeared from most medical school curricula, including counseling, nutrition, exercise therapeutics, homeopathy, botanical medicine, hydrotherapy, and physical therapies. (See Appendix for comparison chart.)

Like any physician, a naturopathic physician takes medical histories, performs physical exams, orders lab tests, and makes diagnoses. A naturopathic doctor differs from other physicians only in how she treats the diagnosed illness, in what she does with the information gathered. A treatment plan may include nutritional counseling, a homeopathic prescription, and a discussion of how a specific exercise program will benefit the patient's health. The discussion may cover job or family pressures and how they are impacting the patient's life. If indicated, an office visit may include some form of physical therapy. Occasionally, a condition requires minor surgery, e.g., removal of skin tags or closure of a laceration. Finally, in certain situations a naturopathic physician may choose to prescribe pharmaceutical drugs.

As a naturopathic physician, I am not completely opposed to the use of drugs and surgery. I do have certain drugs available to me as part of my formulary. For patients with certain conditions, I believe surgery is a viable, even necessary, option. Conventional medicine excels in its treatment of catastrophic conditions, e.g., major bodily injury after a car accident, or removal of large cancerous growths. When the "big guns" are required, conventional medicine responds with reassuring aggression and swiftness. When a body requires ongoing treatment for a chronic illness, or assistance in rebuilding after a major trauma or illness, conventional medicine has little to offer.

Even "simple" acute conditions have few treatments in the conventional medical system. A college friend, recently graduated from conventional medical school, acknowledged his helplessness in treating common colds. "I mean, I don't even know what to do for myself," he confided. "What can I tell my patients?" I was as surprised by his lack of knowledge as I was by his honesty. I can think of at least half a dozen treatments to resolve a cold, and several therapies to abort a cold in its early stages.

In jettisoning the wisdom of classical medicine, the conventional medical system has lost invaluable resources. Gone is the knowledge of supporting the body and working with the healing power innate in the human body. Largely gone is a true understanding of investing in health as a means of prevention. Unfortunately, the big guns of conventional medicine have provided people with a false sense of security. Many people assume that they can continue to eat lifeless food, avoid exercise, smoke, and drink to excess, then be "saved" from illness later in life by the wonders of modern medicine. Half a century after the introduction of the pharmaceutical wonder drugs, we are learning that drug miracles are temporary, not permanent, phenomena. Bacteria and viruses mutate and become resistant to antibiotics. Chemotherapy and anti-hypertensive medications have serious and sometimes irreversible side effects. Such "miracles" exact as many payments as they offer rewards, and the borrowing margin is the health and vitality of our bodies.

Naturopathic medicine relies on the body's innate strength for its miracles. Its wonder drugs are reliable plant and elemental sources that have been used effectively since the dawn of the healing arts.

NATUROPATHIC MEDICAL PHILOSOPHY

Vis Medicatrix Naturae: The Healing Power of Nature

Both our human bodies and the Earth's body have an innate wisdom that governs the cycles of birth, growth, maturation, and decay. Bodily health is supported by moving and living in harmony with these natural cycles. Many healing tools come directly from the Earth. Hydrotherapy, for example, relies on the healing qualities of water. Botanical medicines derive their restorative properties from plants. Mineral, plant, and animal substances provide the foundation for homeopathic medicines. Each of these medications has a native intelligence that interacts with the body's healing wisdom to bring about health, balance, and harmony. Health is a result of balance, which may be maintained by what appear to be destructive forces—e.g., fever or inflammation—that ultimately restore the health and vitality of our bodies (see "Paradigm of Health and Disease," below).

Tolle Causum: Identify and Treat the Cause

Illness does not occur without cause. The body, in its elegant wisdom, always whispers before it shouts. Informed health care means learning to listen to the body and its early warning signs. Body symptoms are metaphors—or, perhaps more accurately, markers—of shifts and changes in life processes. Symptoms usually are the result of the body trying to rebalance itself. Identifying the cause requires seeking the psychic, social, and spiritual roots of the problem, as well as the physical causes of disease. Symptomatic treatment rarely addresses the underlying disturbance. In fact, symptomatic treatment may suppress the illness and make the cause more difficult to identify. Treating the cause requires addressing the body as a whole.

Chinese medicine refers to the treatment principles of *ben* and *biao*, the "roots" and "branches" of disease. The skillful physician learns to differentiate between the deep-seated causes (roots) and the peripheral manifestations (branches) of a disease. "When considering the root (*ben*) and manifestation (*biao*)," writes Maciocia in *The Foundations of Chinese Medicine*, "it is important to understand the connection between the two. They are not separate entities, but two aspects of a contradiction, like *yin* and *yang*. As their names suggest, they are related to one another, just as the roots of a tree are connected to its branches, the former under the ground and invisible, the latter above the ground and visible. The same relation exists between the root of a disease and its clinical manifestations: they are indissolubly related, and they are from two aspects of the same entity."

Treating the cause means addressing the roots of an illness, not just the stems and leaves that symbolize signs and symptoms in the body. The root imbalance may manifest as a group of symptoms. Sometimes several damaged roots manifest as one symptom, e.g., shortness of breath may be a symptom related to several concurrent illnesses such as congestive heart failure, pulmonary edema, chronic bronchitis, and/or emphysema. A guiding principle in both Chinese and naturopathic medicine is "To treat a disease, find the root."

"First Do No Harm"

Classical, natural therapeutics aim to rebalance the body with the least invasive treatments possible. In my practice, I always begin with the simplest treatments (generally dietary changes and hydrotherapy) before adding more complex, and more expensive, treatments. I will prescribe a well-balanced herbal formula before recommending a bag full of supplements. "Doing no harm" also includes implementing therapies that nourish and strengthen the body. Both western and eastern classical medical traditions employ "tonics," herbs and other formulas that strengthen the body. These tonics generally are prescribed after births (for the mother) and after long-term illnesses, and for preventive care. The Chinese, for example, often drink special teas and eat certain foods at the change of each season to prepare the body for new environmental conditions.

Doctor as Teacher

The word *docere* means "to teach." The physician's primary function is to provide information, thus empowering people to regulate their own health. A great deal of time in a naturopathic physician's practice is spent educating patients. Once a patient has applied the information and achieved improved levels of health, the physician serves as a source of further information for emergencies, or as a coach for reaching even higher levels of health.

Unfortunately, some patients do not want such information. They want to be fixed like a car in an auto service center. After spending nearly an hour coaching a patient on diet, exercise changes, and stress reduction, trying to explain why her (mostly junk food) diet was intimately linked with her fatigue, the patient gave me an exasperated look. "Can't you just give me some pills?" she said. "I mean, the last naturopathic physician I went to gave me some tablets, and I felt better as long as I was taking them. Can't you just give me something to take?"

Reluctantly, I prescribed some antioxidants, knowing that I was offering a Band-Aid for a much bigger problem. In addition to poor diet and lack of exercise, the patient worked a very stressful job and nursed her terminally ill mother in the evenings. She was overwhelmed at the prospect of making any significant changes in her life. She wanted her health to improve without changing any of the conditions that were contributing to her illness.

Many people continue to operate in a paradigm engendered by the conventional medical system: "I'm hurting. Give me a pill to take away the pain so I can continue on with my life." The problem with this paradigm is that sometimes the patient's lifestyle is the *cause* of the pain.

Simply taking away the pain with a "magic bullet" will not empower that patient. Even some naturopathic physicians are content to prescribe for quick symptomatic relief and hope the patient will return one day to address the underlying condition.

Perhaps in the situation I have described, I needed to spend more time in the educative process. And perhaps the patient, at this time in her life, was not ready for a medical model that required her participation. Not every patient is interested in health or empowerment. For such patients, drugs and surgery may be valid choices.

Prevention

Preventive care requires studying health as closely as one studies the processes of disease. Most conventional medical practices focus on disease, returning patients from prone to a standing position (crisis intervention). Classical medicine likewise can return patients from prone to standing, and can also help them to walk, run, and, finally dance in their physical forms. Conventional medicine aims for survival; classical medicine aims for optimal health.

True preventive medicine requires making daily investments in our health—eating foods that nourish our bodies, exercising, developing loving relationships and supportive communities, contributing to the health of the Earth. Healthy people live in healthy environments. Preventive medicine means working for clean air, land, and water. Human health is inseparable from the health of the planet.

Treat the Whole Person

The cause of disease is almost always multifactorial; hence, the treatment must be multifaceted. Usually I ask a patient,

"What is going on in your life? Why do think you are ill right now?" Some are surprised. They are not used to having a physician consider anything but physical symptoms and the results of lab tests in the diagnostic work-up. Many already know the cause of their illness. Others need coaching and cajoling to understand that their physical bodies are intimately linked with their mental, emotional, and spiritual lives.

I do not mean to imply that every physical disturbance can be traced to an emotional, mental, or spiritual cause. At one time, I was convinced that all illness was due to an "issue" or "issues" the patient was manifesting through physical illness. Identifying and changing emotional/ mental patterns would resolve the physical illness. Over time, my thinking has changed. Sometimes people do create diseases to work through "issues." Other times people have an iron deficiency because they have an iron deficiency, not because they have some great cosmic lesson to learn. Letting go of the need to find a "metaphysical" cause for every illness has allowed me to be much less judgmental, and much more understanding of the complexities of health and disease. Abandoning my certainty about the causes of disease has provided much more room for the great mystery of health and disease to express itself.

The healing process often causes unresolved wounds from the past to resurface. Such wounding may have occurred on the physical, mental, emotional, or spiritual level. Focusing on healing any aspect of the self can restimulate past hurts as well. The body has enough energy to "clean house"—to bring forth, examine, and discharge past garbage. Clearing emotional pain, for example, may be accompanied by the return of a skin rash that plagued the patient during childhood. Healing the rash may be followed by the realization of an unworkable relationship pattern that he or she is ready to change. The path by which someone returns to wholeness is unique to each individual, although certain patterns of healing may typify that path. The template of healing outlined below is common to both naturopathic and homeopathic medicines:

The Laws of Cure

Healing occurs

- from inside to outside (internal organs first, skin last)
- from top to bottom (from the head region down to the feet)
- from most recent to most distant (recent symptoms recur first, followed by older symptoms—in other words, in reverse chronological order)
- from least important to most important organs

PARADIGM OF HEALTH AND DISEASE

Each healing art operates within a particular framework that elucidates the causes of illness and outlines methods for returning to a state of health. Chapter 2 will explore some of the major healing systems that fall under the umbrella of naturopathic medicine.

Outlined below is a basic paradigm that explains the development of disease from a naturopathic perspective. The model also suggests how to reverse the disease process and return to a state of health.

Keep in mind that a model is not necessarily the "truth." An enlightened teacher once said that we entertain ourselves with models until the truth reveals itself. Although the following paradigm may not represent absolute truth, I

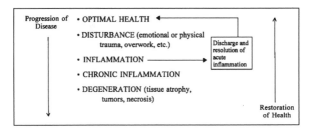

have seen this model function very effectively in clinical practice. The outline provides a simple, elegant understanding of health, illness, and healing that is a major source of guidance for me in my practice.

Most of us begin life in a state of optimal health. Through the course of living, we are exposed to conditions that disturb our equilibrium, that challenge the body beyond its ability to compensate. The body responds by generating inflammation (*rubor*, *dolor*, *calor*, and *tumor*—redness, pain, heat, and swelling). Fever is one of the most common inflammatory responses.

Inflammation is the body's way of discharging a disturbance from the body. If the body is allowed to complete the inflammatory response, the disturbance is discharged, and the body returns to optimal health:

Optimal Health→Disturbance→Inflammation→
Discharge→Optimal Health

Natural therapeutics, when properly applied, can speed up the discharge phase and hasten the return to health. Unfortunately, most people attempt to stop the inflammatory response before it has a chance to discharge the disturbance from the body. Stopping or suppressing the inflammation can drive the disturbance deeper into the body, causing chronic irritation. If chronic irritation continues long enough, the body tissues begin to degenerate (atrophy, tumors, necrosis).

Optimal Health→Disturbance→Inflammation→Suppression→
Chronic Inflammation→Tissue degeneration

A classic example of suppression, recognized by conventional as well as naturopathic medicine, is applying cortisone cream to eczema rashes. Cortisone stops inflammation by suppressing the activity of the immune system. Patients with eczema who apply cortisone creams often notice that asthma develops (or worsens) as the eczema clears. In essence, the cortisone cream suppresses the eczema and drives the inflammation deeper into the body, in this case to the lungs. Patients often notice that, as their asthma improves, the eczema returns—the body has strengthened to the point of pushing the inflammation to the surface (skin) once again (see the "Laws of Cure," above). They reapply the cortisone cream, the eczema improves, and the asthma worsens. This chronic cycle of suppression and improvement may continue for years before the body becomes too weary to push the inflammation to the surface any longer. At that point, the eczema diminishes to a low-grade irritation as the asthma becomes a more deep-seated, chronic condition.

Natural therapeutics, when improperly applied, can also cause suppression of inflammation and irritation. Although suppression is less likely with natural therapeutics, a practitioner of hydrotherapy, herbs, and homeopathics must be mindful of his or her prescriptions and watch carefully for any signs of suppression. In the example given above, asthma is a "chronic irritation" of the lung tissue caused by suppressing a surface irritation. From a naturopathic perspective, the surface irritation (eczema) is a less serious condition than chronic inflammation in a vital organ (asthma). If the chronic inflammation continues long enough, degeneration of tissues will occur.

Generally the body will not develop measurable signs of damage until the disease has reached the "chronic inflammation" or "degeneration" level. Taking a biopsy of an acutely infected sinus, for example, and examining the tissue under a microscope usually will not reveal major tissue changes. A chronically infected sinus, however, will show signs of irritation at the cellular level. Long-term irritation may cause degeneration of the tissues. Necrosis is a late-stage manifestation of tissue degeneration.

The model for returning to health is a reversal of the disease process.

Degeneration→Chronic Inflammation→Inflammation→
Discharge→Optimal Health

From a naturopathic perspective, the healing process is stimulated first through the digestive system, by two central methods—proper nutrition and hydrotherapy. The digestive system is absolutely essential for the regeneration of any body tissue. The alimentary tract is responsible for absorption of all nutrients and disposal of most wastes in the body. If the digestive system is functioning optimally, the body has a fighting chance of receiving all the nutrition available in the food we eat, and disposing of all the wastes generated by the body during the natural processes of maintenance and repair.

Constitutional hydrotherapy—a specific hydrotherapy treatment designed to stimulate the immune system and increase circulation in the digestive system—is the simplest, most powerful, least expensive method to support healing of the digestive tract. (See "Hydrotherapy" section of Chapter 2.)

Dietary changes and constitutional-hydrotherapy treatments also stimulate something that our current medical terminology has no tool to measure—the body's own innate healing ability. As the body strengthens, the disease process begins to reverse itself. Degeneration improves to the level of chronic irritation, and then chronic irritation becomes acute—the body finally has enough energy to "clean house," to bring the acute inflammation that was suppressed back to the surface. Often the acute inflammation returns in the form of a low-grade fever, or a cold or flu-like illness, that lasts for a couple of days. Sometimes the housecleaning, also referred to as the "healing crisis," manifests as the return of an old illness. In contrast to earlier episodes, however, the healing crisis usually is much briefer and less intense than the original occurrence.

If allowed to run its course, the acute inflammation allows the body to discharge the original disturbance, and the body returns once again to a state of optimal health. When the body finally mounts an acute inflammation after a long, chronic illness, remember that the inflammation must be allowed to run its course without any further suppression (e.g., no cortisone or aspirin).

In addition to nutrition and hydrotherapy, many other treatments stimulate the body's innate healing ability. Homeopathy, botanical medicines, stress reduction, acupuncture, and physical therapies all may support the body in its healing journey. Inner work, meditation, and counseling address the roots of some illnesses. Choosing a particular modality requires both skill and intuition—a practitioner needs a solid knowledge of his or her subject, and a well-honed intuition to select the method or methods that will most benefit a patient. Often I tell patients that we will be doing some "detective work," discovering what treatments will be most catalytic for them. Of course, the response depends in part on the skill of the practitioner, and on his or her ability to utilize a particular healing tool.

This marriage of knowledge and intuition is paramount for application of these principles at home. Learn everything you can about the modalities you find most useful, or to which you feel most drawn. Consult local practitioners, read, and study. Practice what you are learning. Information becomes living knowledge when you apply the information in your life. Learn to listen to your intuition, the "natural intelligence" that guides the application of knowledge. Remember that each person is different, and that what affects one person may not affect another. As you become more familiar with your own and your family's bodies, you will make better and better selections based on your healing knowledge.

Chapter Two
Therapies

So, you've decided to improve your health and reap the rewards of increased energy, flexibility, concentration, and creativity. You've begun to walk down the aisles of the whole-foods store and the public library searching for resources to help you fulfill your dreams of improved health.

Choosing a therapeutic approach can be the most exciting, frustrating, rewarding, and baffling search for anyone interested in the healing arts. Take a deep breath. Know that over time you probably will explore several healing modalities. Some paths will reward you; others will meander or dead-end before you decide to explore other byways.

Each healing modality has an important role to play. The art of working with natural therapeutics is matching your needs with the natural intelligence invested in each therapeutic method. What works well for you may be anathema for a neighbor or your spouse. Respect your differences. What works well for one person may not necessarily work for another. Your body also may respond to different methods at different times—keep listening to your body's needs and note its responses over time.

If you are fortunate to have a naturopathic physician in your community, you may be able to bypass some of the trial-and-error tactics involved in discovering the therapeutics that work best for you. Together with your naturopathic physician you can do the "detective work" needed to identify the most supportive treatment methods for you. You also will benefit from his or her expertise in applying the most appropriate healing modalities in your specific situation. To become a gifted homeopathic prescriber, for example, may require a lifetime of study. You can bypass some of the frustration of investing in books and remedies and obtaining marginal results by working with someone who already has studied a particular modality. Best of all, find a physician who offers classes in how to apply natural therapeutics in your daily life.

The following is an outline of the chief healing modalities employed by naturopathic physicians, including brief descriptions of other major systems of medicine that share a common philosophy with naturopathic medicine. When working with a new patient, I consider potential treatments in a particular order, based on what I know of how the body heals. The following list of therapeutics reflects that order. In addition to describing the therapy, I've included information on how and when to consider using a specific treatment. My hope is that this information will assist you in deciding when to choose a particular treatment.

MIND, EMOTION, SPIRIT

No amount of physical therapy or herbs can take the place of companionship in the life of a lonely person. The "perfect" acupuncture treatment cannot compensate for a soul-draining job or an emotionally toxic home environment. In these and other situations, therapeutic methods offer, at best, a means of supporting someone until he or she is ready to make the kinds of life changes that will engender overall health.

I hesitate to place this at the top of the list, again for fear of falling into the trap of identifying a "spiritual imbalance" or "emotional issue" at the root of every illness. Keep in mind that people with a profound spiritual connection and a rich, positive emotional life still can manifest disease in their bodies. Too many malnourished, overworked women (and sometimes men) have been told that their illnesses are in their heads, that they should quit complaining and get on with their lives. Clearly, their illnesses are *not* all in their heads. Recovery involves the physical body as well as the patient's mental or emotional state.

When illness develops, a simple way of utilizing the therapy of mind, emotions, and spirit is to ask yourself the following questions:

- What is going on in my life now?
- What are the biggest concerns—the major stressors—in my life now?
- Am I working too much? Too little? Does my work bring me satisfaction?
- Is my lifestyle sustainable, i.e., can I complete everything I need to complete and still remain healthy?
- Are my relationships supporting me? Am I investing time and attention in the major relationships in my life?

Twylah Nitsch, a Seneca elder, poses the following questions:

- Am I happy with what I'm doing?
- Is what I'm doing adding to the confusion?
- What am I doing to bring about peace and contentment?
- How will I be remembered when I'm gone?

Keep in mind that these questions are a *beginning*. They are meant to invoke insight, not provide fodder for self-destructive thoughts (i.e., don't beat yourself up if you discover some challenging areas). Illnesses can offer the opportunity to slow down and reevaluate our lives, to make new choices based on our greatest dreams, our deepest joys.

These questions may serve as a good reality check as well. When humans endure a certain intensity or number of stresses, the body is more likely to develop an illness. One of my current patients has struggled with depression for almost three years. Reviewing her life shortly before the onset of the depression provided some obvious clues about the cause of her depression: within the space of six months, she lost five family members and two close friends. Further history revealed that she was adopted and shared a pattern common to many adopted children—she felt profoundly abandoned when significant people exited from her life. We continue to pursue supportive therapies in conjunction with counseling, with an understanding that true healing probably will require deep emotional work to resolve her primary experience of loss and abandonment.

NUTRITION

A healthy digestive system is vital to overall health. The digestive system is responsible for the absorption of the majority of our nutrients and for the removal of most waste from the body. Even the most nutritious food and the best supplements will not be fully utilized if the digestive system is unable to absorb the nutrients and dispose of waste.

The body has two nervous systems running simultaneously, the sympathetic and parasympathetic. They both function at all times, but one always predominates. When the sympathetic nervous system is more active, the body is in "fight or flight" mode, geared up to protect us from danger. The body responds to outside stress in the same way whether the "predator" is a hungry tiger or an irritated boss. Norepinephrine (adrenalin) dumps into the bloodstream, increasing the heart and respiratory rates. The vascular system responds by shunting blood away from the internal organs toward the peripheral muscles to prepare for quick movement. The digestive system begins to "shut down" with reduced gastric secretions and peristalsis.

Many people in today's culture live continuously on low on levels of adrenalin, with the sympathetic nervous system predominating. In this situation, the digestive system receives very little blood flow. Food sits in the digestive tract for long periods of time without adequate supplies of gastric juices to digest it. The digestive tract cannot adequately absorb nutrients or expel wastes.

The parasympathetic nervous system predominates when we are relaxed, favoring regeneration of body tissues and increased activity in the digestive tract. You may have noticed that your stomach and intestines gurgle when you are relaxed and happy. This gurgling (not to be confused with the growls of hunger) is a good sign, indicating that the digestive system is working well.

If the digestive system is not functioning optimally, even the healthiest foods and the most potent nutritional supplements will not be utilized fully by the body. In addition, one nutritionist noted that Americans have the most expensive urine in the world: we swallow pills that cannot be utilized by the body because the digestive system has a difficult time breaking down the pills. The body can use only a certain amount of water-soluble vitamins at any one time; within a short period, unused vitamins are dumped into the urine for removal.

Proper nutrition starts with identifying any foods that may cause irritation in the digestive tract. Many lab tests exist to identify food allergies, irritants, and sensitivities. One such test checks for constitutional food intolerances—foods the body fundamentally does not digest well. If the body is repeatedly exposed to these foods over a long period of time, the gut becomes irritated. Eventually the irritation causes a breakdown of the intestinal mucosa. "Leaky gut" syndrome develops, and larger molecules of food cross the gut mucosa. The immune system, unused to seeing these large molecules, may develop antibodies to fight the presumed "foreign" invaders.

Avoiding food allergens and sensitivities can help to resolve innumerable symptoms; however, simply avoiding foods will not cause the gut to heal, nor will it help to identify the *primary* foods that caused the gut disturbance in the first place. Identifying constitutional food intolerances satisfies one part of the equation—removing the root cause of irritation in the gut. In addition to taking away the primary disturbance, the body requires support to encourage regeneration of healthy gut mucosa.

Constitutional hydrotherapy is the simplest, most powerful method to support healing of the digestive tract. See the following "Hydrotherapy" section for specific instructions for the constitutional hydrotherapy treatment.

Basic Guidelines for Better Nutrition

1. Eat foods as close as possible to their natural state. A baked potato, for example, contains more nutrition (and fewer additives) than potato chips. Whole, fresh apples contain more roughage and nutrients than apple juice.

27

2. Eat local foods, which generally contain the nutrients that are best for the local population. In the Pacific Northwest, for example, wild salmon have high levels of essential fatty acids, which help prevent hormonal swings associated with "seasonal affective disorder," a common malady in Oregon and Washington. Eating local foods also reduces fossil fuel consumption by eliminating the need to truck or fly foods long distances.

3. Buy organic foods. Recent studies show that organic foods have at least 70 percent more nutrients than their conventionally grown counterparts. In addition, organic foods are free of petroleum-based pesticides and herbicides. The chemical residues tend to concentrate in our reproductive organs and fatty tissues, causing decreased fertility, breast cancer, and a host of other degenerative diseases. In the long run, organic agriculture contributes to soil fertility and overall ecosystem health, while reducing our reliance on fossil fuels.

4. Choose foods low on the food chain. In other words, choose grains, legumes, and vegetables more frequently than fish or meat. The following are general guidelines for nutrition based on calorie intake. Keep in mind, however, that each individual varies radically in her or his nutritional needs.

   - 70 percent grains and legumes
   - 20 percent fruits and vegetables
   - 10 percent meat, cheese, eggs, tofu, and other concentrated protein sources

Most Americans eat far too much concentrated protein. The processing of excess protein metabolites by the kidneys can weaken organ function over a period of time. All food sources, including plant foods, contain protein. The World Health Organization recommends eating 50 grams of protein per day, with increased amounts for pregnant or lactating women.

5. Ideal fat content in the diet is 10–15 percent of the daily caloric intake. The type of fat or oil is as important as the quantity. Altered fats (rancid or hydrogenated fats and oils) should be eliminated entirely from the diet. These include margarines and shortenings, whether they are used fresh, or included in processed and deep-fried foods. Keep saturated animal fats to a minimum. Include cold-pressed, properly stored oils in your daily diet. Keep all oils, including olive oil, in the refrigerator: heat, light, and air cause oils to become rancid.

6. Take time to chew. Some sources recommend chewing every bite of food as many as fifty times. This first step in the digestive process grinds food into smaller pieces and mixes saliva with the food. Saliva contains many enzymes that begin the process of carbohydrate digestion before the food ever leaves the mouth. Following this simple advice can eliminate a host of digestive complaints.

HYDROTHERAPY

Earth is a water planet, bestowed with a blue-green vastness of liquid life. Our bodies are 70 percent water—we left the amniotic support of the sea by learning to contain it within our skin. Humans can survive for weeks without food. Without water, we perish within days, even hours in an arid desert climate.

For thousands of years water has been used to treat disease and trauma, with various revivals punctuating its long history. At his mountain sanitarium, Vincent Priessnitz (1799–1852) championed the most recent European rediscovery of water's healing properties. In the United States, John Harvey Kellogg, M.D. (1852–1943) was a major proponent of water cures. His Battle Creek Sanitarium combined water treatments with sine-wave, massage, and dietary therapies. (His method of pressing whole grains into "flakes" survives today in the Kellogg cereal industry.) Kellogg kept meticulous records and conducted scientific research in his sanitarium. The data gathered became the foundation for *Rational Hydrotherapy* (1901), still the definitive textbook on the subject.

Hydrotherapy involves the use of hot and cold water in specific treatments to stimulate the immune system and alter blood circulation to particular areas of the body. Outlined below are five specific hydrotherapy treatments that can be used to treat a wide range of conditions.

GENERAL CAUTION: Diabetic patients should never apply heat to the feet. This also applies to anyone with compromised circulation in the extremities (e.g., Raynaud's Syndrome). Instead, apply a large fomentation (towels wrung out in very warm water) to the groin area.

Constitutional Hydrotherapy Treatment

The constitutional hydrotherapy treatment increases immune-system function, improves digestion, and promotes detoxification. It can be used to treat almost any acute or chronic condition. In a trained hydrotherapist's clinic, the treatment would include the use of a sine-wave machine to further stimulate the digestive tract. The following instructions are for home application.

When not to apply this treatment: in acute cases of asthma, acute bladder infection, or low body temperature (below 97°F oral temperature). Be careful to avoid drafts or chills during the treatment. Apply a hot-water bottle to the feet and add more blankets if you feel chilly.

Equipment
- shower or bath
- one towel
- two blankets
- one sheet

Directions
1. Spread the blankets lengthwise on a bed with the sheet over them.
2. Wet the towel with cold water and wring out excess water. The towel should be damp, not dripping.
3. Take a hot bath or shower, as hot as you can comfortably stand it, for 5–10 minutes. You should feel warm after the bath or shower; if not, postpone the treatment until you are feeling warmer.
4. Get out of the shower and dry off.
5. Wrap the cold towel all the way around your trunk.
6. Lie down on the blankets and sheet prepared earlier.
7. Wrap the sheets and blankets snugly around you.
8. Sleep, rest, meditate, or listen to quiet music for 25–30 minutes, or until your body has warmed the toweling.

NOTE: The greater the contrast between hot and cold applications, the stronger the treatment. You can increase the effect of the treatment by placing the cold, wet towel in the freezer for 5–10 minutes before applying.

Salt-Water Lavage and Gargle

This treatment helps to eliminate excessive mucous from the nose and throat. Salt water soothes inflamed mucosal tissue *and* acts as an anti-microbial. Viruses and bacteria cannot survive in a concentrated saline solution. The difference in osmotic pressure between the salt solution and their own cellular-fluid concentration causes the viruses and bacteria literally to explode.

Begin gargling with salt water at the first sign of a sore throat. Repeat every 3–4 hours until the symptoms resolve. Use the nasal lavage technique when nasal congestion develops, or after exposure to irritating inhalants (e.g., dust, air pollution, mold).

Equipment
- tall glass or large cup
- water, as warm as you can comfortably tolerate
- 1–2 teaspoons of sea salt (non-iodized)

Directions
1. Add sea salt to glass of warm water.
2. For gargle, take one mouthful of salt water at a time. Some physicians recommend swallowing the salt water after gargling. Do not swallow the salt water if you have hypertension or diabetes.
3. For nasal lavage, pour salt water into your cupped hand. Gently inhale the salt water, then gently blow the water from the nostrils. This is best done over a sink. At the end of the treatment, be sure to blow any excess water from the nose. You may notice increased nasal and sinus drainage after the treatment.

NOTE: Too much or too little salt or cool water may cause nasal tingling and discomfort. Adjust the water temperature or amount of salt if you experience nasal discomfort.

Wet-socks Treatment

This simple, powerful treatment stimulates the production and activity of white blood cells and draws congestion away from the upper body. The wet-socks treatment speeds resolution of an upper-respiratory infection. If used when the very first symptoms begin, the treatment can even abort a cold.

Equipment
- foot bath (a plastic dishpan works well, or sit on the edge of a bathtub and soak feet in hot, shallow water)
- towel
- one pair of cotton ankle-high socks
- one pair of wool socks

Directions
1. Soak feet in water as hot as you can comfortably tolerate for 5–10 minutes. Add more hot water if necessary.
2. Dry feet.
3. Wet cotton socks in cold tap water. Wring out thoroughly. (Socks should be damp, not dripping.)
4. Get in bed. Put on the damp cotton socks. Immediately cover with the wool socks.
5. Go to sleep.

NOTE: This treatment is best done right before bedtime. In most cases, the socks will be dry by morning.

Hot Foot Bath

A hot foot bath can treat a wide variety of ailments, from simple tension headaches, to upper-respiratory infections, to menstrual cramps.

Equipment
- plastic dishpan, tub, or bowl large enough to soak the feet
- towel for drying feet

Directions
1. Fill the pan with enough water to cover the ankles. The water should be as hot as you can comfortably stand it.
2. Soak the feet for 5–10 minutes maximum. More than ten minutes of heat exposure promotes congestion more than circulation.

For a more powerful treatment, alternate between hot-water and cold-water baths.

1. Soak the feet in hot water for five minutes.
2. Soak the feet in cold water for one minute.
3. Repeat this cycle at least three times.
4. Always end with cold water.

Alternating Hot and Cold Applications

Alternating hot and cold applications to a local area increases circulation and decreases congestion. From a Chinese perspective, congestion or "stagnation" causes pain. This simple method can be employed to reduce pain and swelling associated with acute injuries, ear infections, headaches, and other conditions.

In general, the greater the contrast in temperature between the hot and cold applications, the stronger the treatment. For children, the elderly, and severely debilitated people (e.g., terminal cancer, late stages of AIDS or emphysema), moderate the temperature extremes.

Equipment
- two towels
- a large pan of hot water, or a microwave

- a pan of cold water, with ice cubes (if tolerated)
- plastic sheet (or an old shower curtain), if needed to protect bedding

Directions

1. Always begin with a 3–5-minute hot application. This can be a towel wrung out in hot water (as hot as you can stand it) or a wetted towel placed in a microwave for 3–4 minutes. If the towel is too hot, shake it back and forth for a couple of moments—towels cool quickly. Apply the towel to the affected area.
2. Apply a cold application (towel wrung out in cold tap water or ice water) to the affected area for one minute.
3. Repeat this cycle at least three times.
4. Always end with a cold application.

General Advice

- Make sure an area is warm before applying a cold towel. If someone is severely chilled, or if the body temperature is below 98°F, warm the body with a hot bath or shower before applying cold towels.
- For acute earaches, a 40-watt light bulb can be substituted for a hot, wet towel. Sit 6–8 inches away from the light bulb, close enough to feel heat, but not close enough to burn the skin. To reduce pain associated with earache, use heat alone for up to 30 minutes.
- A hot-water bottle can substitute for a hot, wet towel.
- For a small area, frozen peas in a plastic bag can be substituted for a cold, wet towel.

BOTANICAL MEDICINE

The plant realm provides an astounding array of medicines. Botanical medicines, or herbs, are available in several forms.

Consider growing your own medicinal herbs—you will learn much more about their healing properties, and you will have a steady supply of medicines.

Outlined below are some basic preparation techniques and dosage instructions. Please follow the recommended dosages for the different types of herbs to achieve maximum benefit while minimizing potential side effects from overdosage.

A Note on Dosages

The following is a general rule of thumb for dosing herbs:

- For acute illnesses, take two dropperfuls of tincture, or two capsules of dried herb, every 2–4 hours, depending on the severity of the condition.
- *Six years old*: take half the adult dosage (i.e., one dropperful every 2–4 hours)
- *Three years old*: take one-fourth the adult dosage.
- *One year old*: take one-sixth the adult dosage.

A Few Definitions

Infusion (steeped tea): For leafy herbs, use one ounce of herbs per pint of water. Bring water to a boil and pour over the herbs. Steep for 10–15 minutes, strain, and drink.

Decoction (simmered tea): Roots, berries, and thick leaves require more than infusing to release the healing constituents of the plant. Bring a pint of water to a boil, then add two tablespoons of dried herb to the water. Simmer for 10–15 minutes. If you are adding leaves to the herbal formula, add them to the decoction after simmering, remove the pan from the burner, and allow the herbs to steep for another ten minutes.

Tincture: Tinctures are made by soaking herbs in a solvent—generally food-grade alcohol or vinegar—to produce a concentrated herbal medicine. The constituents released, which will vary depending on the solvent and the herb, are similar to those found in botanical infusions and decoctions, albeit in a more concentrated form.

Essential Oils

Essential oils are extremely concentrated herbal preparations. An ounce of essential oil represents several pounds of dried plant material. Use the oils respectfully.

Inhalations: Steam inhalations are very effective for breaking up lung and sinus congestion. Steam also deep-cleans the skin. Pour boiling water into a large bowl or pan. Add two or three drops of essential oil. Make a "tent" by draping a towel over the head and edges of the basin. Lean over the hot water and inhale the steam. End the treatment by rinsing the face with cold water.

Internal use: For stomach upset, add one drop of essential oil of peppermint to a glass of warm water. Never take more than one or two drops of essential oil internally. Some essential oils (e.g., sandalwood) are toxic and should never be taken internally.

External use: Add four to five drops of essential oil to a cup of vegetable oil for a soothing massage or after-bath oil. Oils of peppermint, eucalyptus, clove, and/or tea tree added to vegetable oil or petroleum jelly make a soothing chest rub for coughs and colds. If the essential oil causes a skin rash even when diluted in vegetable oil, discontinue use.

CAUTION: Applying essential oils directly to the skin can cause irritation and skin rash. Never apply to the area around the eyes or genitals, where essential oils can cause tissue damage.

Baths

The skin and muscles especially benefit from herbal baths. Place herbs in a soft, loosely woven cloth (muslin is ideal), gather the edges in at the center, and tie with a string or ribbon. Tie the herbal pouch below the water spigot so that warm bath water runs through it as you fill the tub. *Alternate method:* steep herbs as for an herbal infusion and add the strained tea to the bath water.

Granules

Chinese herbs are sometimes prepared in granular form. The granules are made from evaporated herbal teas.

Basic Herbs For the Home Medicine Chest

Alfalfa (*Medicago sativa*) leaves—Alfalfa has an overall tonifying effect on the body, making it an ideal herb to help rebuild after a major illness. Encourages healthy teeth and gum tissue.

Chamomile (*Matricaria chamomila*) flowers—Chamomile contains high levels of calcium, making it an excellent nerve and muscle relaxant. Chamomile soothes upset stomach, and encourages sleep if taken 1–2 hours before bedtime.

Dandelion (*Taraxacum officinalis*) root and leaf—Dandelion leaf acts as a diuretic, potent enough to affect even congestive heart failure. Dandelion root is a liver tonic, increasing bile production and encouraging detoxification.

Echinacea (*Echinacea angustafolia* or *purpurea*) flowers— Echinacea's antimicrobial action is excellent for upper-respiratory infections. As a general immune stimulant, echinacea increases white blood cell activity.

Ginger (*Zingiber officinalis*) root—Ginger is a warming carminative, soothing digestive function. Ginger also acts as a diaphoretic, inducing sweating.

Goldenseal (*Hydrastis canadensis*) root—Goldenseal is antimicrobial and tonic for both the digestive and circulatory systems. Helpful for chronic stomach problems, sinusitis, colds, and coughs.

NOTE: Goldenseal also kills helpful intestinal bacteria. After taking a course of goldenseal, encourage repopulation of normal gut flora by eating fresh sauerkraut, yogurt, kefir, or Korean *kim chee* (cabbage pickled in garlic and chile).

Mint (*Mentha piperita*) leaves and essential oil—Mint leaves can be brewed into a tea for upset stomach, or taken at the beginning of a cold. One or two drops of essential oil in a bowl of hot water makes a wonderful vapor inhalation for a cough or cold. Mint has the ability to increase oxygenation, thereby helping to stop bacterial and viral lung infections.

Nettles (*Urtica urens*) leaves—Nettle leaves are a powerful spring tonic, particularly beneficial for the kidneys.

Oatstraw (*Avena sativa*) straw and seed chaff—Oatstraw is soothing and nourishing for the nerves. Also excellent for stress, anxiety, and mild insomnia.

Red raspberry leaf (*Rubus ideus*) leaves—This uterine tonic helps normalize menstrual periods and supports uterine tone during pregnancy.

Yarrow (*Achillea millefolium*) flowers—Yarrow stanches bleeding and acts as a diaphoretic, inducing sweating and mild temperature elevation. As a urinary antiseptic, yarrow can help stop urinary-tract infections if taken in the early stages.

NOTE: All leafy herbs (e.g., mint leaves) should be replaced annually. If kept longer, the herbs lose their essential oils and other healing constituents. Root herbs may be kept for two seasons if stored in a cool, dry place.

HOMEOPATHIC MEDICINE

Homeopathy, which literally means "study of similars," is a medical science that shares a common healing philosophy with naturopathic medicine. Both aim to stimulate the body's innate healing capacity to bring about a "cure." Developed by Samuel Hahnemann, a late-18th-century German physician, the science of homeopathy grew out of Hahnemann's years of medical-text translations. Discouraged by the medical practices of his day, Hahnemann turned to translating medical texts in part to support his large family, and also in hopes of discovering, or rediscovering, certain universal laws of healing that seemed to be missing in contemporary medical practice.

While translating a *materia medica*, Hahnemann noted an explanation that quinine cured malaria because of its astringent properties. To test the assertion, Hahnemann took four drams (one-half ounce), or about fifteen doses, of quinine every morning and evening. Within four days he developed the symptoms of malaria in his formerly healthy body. When Hahnemann stopped taking the quinine, the symptoms disappeared.

With this experiment, Hahnemann confirmed the "law of similars," an ancient healing principle of using like to cure like. In other words, a substance that produces symptoms in a healthy person can be used to treat the same symptoms in an ailing person. Hahnemann—and, later, a large following of students—began a series of experiments to test the effects of various plant and mineral extracts on healthy subjects. Hahnemann himself tested and meticulously recorded the effects of many substances before his death in 1843 at the age of eighty-eight.

During his years of research, Hahnemann discovered another basic truth: the more dilute the medicine, the more potent its effect. His discovery ran contrary to the practices of his day, an era when doctors used large doses of mercury, sulfur, coal oil, and other toxic compounds to produce violent, cathartic effects in the body.

Homeopathic remedies are prepared by diluting one drop of base tincture, prepared from the whole plant, in either ten ("x" potencies) or 100 ("c" potencies) drops of water. This mixture is "secussed" (banged or shaken a specific number of times) to potentize the remedy. Next, one drop of the 1x (1:10) or 1c (1:100) solution is placed in a vial with another ten or 100 drops of water. The process is repeated until the solution is the desired potency, or dilution.

Many physicians have dismissed the effects of homeopathic remedies, declaring them placebos. Voluminous clinical studies, however, have demonstrated the efficacy of homeopathic medicines. Recent double-blind research also conclusively demonstrates the effectiveness of homeopathic remedies in treating particular diseases.

Despite positive test results, all double-blind studies of homeopathic treatments share a common weakness: the same homeopathic remedy is given to different subjects suffering with the same disease. In contrast to this procedure, the homeopathic method of prescribing involves assessing the complete symptom picture and choosing a remedy that best suits the individual. One person with a cold, for example, may have severe chills, sensitivity to light, and extreme irritability, while another patient reports having a fever, desiring cold air, and wanting company to console her. For the first patient, the homeopath might prescribe *Nux vomica*; for the second, *Pulsatilla*. In a double-blind study, she would be required to give both patients the same remedy.

Using a double-blind study to test homeopathic medicines is like using a yardstick to measure the pitch of a sound— the instrument is inappropriate for the task. The homeopath's great strength is his or her ability to focus first on the human being and secondarily on the disease.

General Guidelines for Using Homeopathic Medicines for Home Care

- Prescribe the remedy for the specific symptom picture presented, not for the disease (see above).
- The more dilute the medicine, the more potent its effect (i.e., a 30c remedy is stronger than a 12c remedy).
- Homeopathic prescriptions can be made on an acute or a constitutional basis. A constitutional prescription requires a long interview process (1–2 hours) to create a complete picture of the person desiring a remedy. For acute prescriptions, only major symptoms associated with the current ailment are considered.
- Store homeopathic medicines in a cool, dry place away from strong-smelling substances, especially mint, menthol, and camphor. Homeopathic medicines will remain potent for

decades if stored properly. An expiration date is stamped on homeopathic remedies to satisfy FDA regulations.

How To Take Homeopathic Remedies

- One dose of a homeopathic remedy equals three pellets dissolved under the tongue. For liquid preparations, one dose equals three drops under the tongue.
- The effect of a homeopathic remedy is determined by how often you take a dose, not by how many pellets you take. Swallowing three pellets of a homeopathic remedy, for example, is as effective as swallowing fifty. If a child swallows an entire bottle of homeopathic pills, he or she has taken just one dose of the remedy and ordinarily will suffer no ill effects.
- To increase the effect of a remedy, take it more often, e.g., every 2–3 hours during the worst stages of an acute illness.
- When you take a homeopathic remedy for an acute condition, one of four things will happen:
  1. You choose the correct remedy and begin to feel better.
  2. You choose the correct remedy and have an "aggravation" of symptoms. The body, in essence, is preparing to throw off whatever has been irritating it. Someone with a cold, for example, may go through a period of increased nasal discharge and sneezing. For an acute illness, you may feel worse for a short time (usually 3–4 hours), then begin to feel better.
  3. You choose the wrong remedy, have an aggravation of symptoms, but do not feel better after 3–4 hours.
  4. You choose the wrong remedy and nothing happens.
- Stop taking the remedy when you notice improvement.
- Repeat a dose of the same remedy if you notice the symptoms worsening again.

- During the same illness, always repeat the last remedy that caused improvement before trying another remedy. This does not apply to the return of an illness after a significant period of time. For example, someone with a cold early in the autumn may improve with homeopathic *Gelsemium*, while her post-holiday cold in January responds to *Nux vomica*.
- During the course of an acute illness, you may need more than one remedy. The homeopathic prescription changes as the symptom picture changes.
- Avoid using coffee, cola, black tea, mint, menthol, camphor, or strong perfumes while taking homeopathic medicines. These substances can overpower the action of the remedies.

Choosing the Correct Potency

There are as many theories about choosing potencies as there are homeopaths. Below are some of the generally agreed-upon principles for choosing a potency. Some of the information may seem contradictory, and herein lies the art of prescribing homeopathic remedies—knowing when to apply which principle.

Most homeopathic first-aid kits come in 30x or 30c potencies. This is a good mid-range potency with which to begin. Most health-food stores only sell up to 30c potencies. Higher potencies generally require a physician's prescription.

- Young, old, or weakened patients generally respond best to lower potencies (6c or 12c). Their bodies do not need, and sometimes cannot handle, strong stimulation.
- The more physical the symptoms, the lower the dosage. For example, a patient with a sprained ankle would respond better to a lower dosage than a patient suffering with severe depression.

- The more overlap between the overall remedy picture and the patient's symptoms, the higher the dosage. Few patients match every symptom associated with a remedy.
- The more acute or severe an ailment, the higher the potency you should administer and the more often you can repeat a remedy. After a car accident, for example, you may administer 200c *Arnica* (very specific for trauma, bruising, and shock) every fifteen minutes. In contrast, a nagging dry cough at the end of a cold may require two doses of 30c *Spongia* per day.

PHYSICAL THERAPIES

Physical therapies include a broad range of techniques and therapeutic approaches. Again, different patients respond best to different techniques. Therapies range from osseous (bone) manipulation and deep-tissue work, to more subtle approaches such as cranio-sacral or Bowen work. The therapies generally address musculoskeletal ailments, although the chiropractic profession has demonstrated quite definitively that a wide range of acute and chronic internal conditions will respond to osseous manipulation.

CHINESE MEDICINE

Balance is the hallmark of Chinese medicine. In a state of health, our bodies are constantly shifting, elegantly balanced organisms. "Balance" by no means implies "static" within the Chinese healing paradigm. A healthy body constantly shifts and changes to maintain a dynamic state of equilibrium. The Chinese refer to the balance of *yin* and *yang*, which encompasses all of the opposites one could imagine—e.g., light/dark, hot/cold, dry/wet, interior/exterior. The Chinese understand that an extreme of any one condition inevitably leads back to its opposite, like the snake curling to bite its own tail. The classic yin/yang symbol contains a spot of light within the dark half, and a spot of dark within the light half, hinting at the understanding that each condition or quality carries the seed of its opposite within itself.

Traditional Chinese medicine aims to address the whole person. Like naturopathic physicians, a practitioner of Chinese medicine will ask questions about a person's constitution, lifestyle patterns, and general physical symptoms. This information allows the practitioner to identify patterns of health or imbalance. Such patterns, or "syndrome pictures," guide the practitioner to the most supportive treatments for a particular patient, treatments that will help restore the balance of the body so that it can return to optimal health.

Traditional Chinese medicine includes four major treatment areas: acupuncture, Chinese herbs, *tui na* (body work), and *qi gong* (movement and meditation). An office visit might include one or more of these four major treatment methods.

"Five Elements" is another branch of Chinese medicine currently practiced in the United States. Practitioners diagnose the relationships between earth, fire, water, air, and metal in the body. Each of these elements relates to the others in a complex, synergistic pattern. The Five Elements practitioner aims to rebalance the five elements and thus restore health to the body.

NOTE: Chinese medicine often describes conditions more poetically than does our objective Western medical terminology. A Chinese medical practitioner, for example, might diagnose someone with "blood deficiency." The patient does not necessarily have a blood imbalance that would show up on a blood test (e.g., anemia), but rather a qualitative reduction of the blood's moistening, cooling properties that might manifest as dry skin and hair. The Chinese also refer to "external pernicious influences" (EPI's) as a cause of disease. These external forces—such as heat, cold, wind, and damp—can enter the body and cause acute illnesses. A common cold with sore throat and headache, for example, might be diagnosed as an invasion of wind and heat.

Acupuncture

Acupuncture works with the body's own energy currents, which are measurable as electromagnetic forces. This magnetic force, or "river of energy, " follows predictable patterns in the body. Chinese practitioners, after centuries of study and observation, have mapped these currents of energy and designated them as "meridians" correlated to particular organs and systems in the body.

Acupuncture helps to direct the energy flow, or *qi*, through the meridians. Very thin needles inserted into "points" on the body help redirect areas of pooled energy ("stagnation") and encourage *qi* to flow into areas that are deficient or undernourished. Ultimately, the acupuncture needles help to rebalance the body's electromagnetic currents, thereby supporting the internal organs and all the body's physiological systems. Redirecting the body's energy currents through acupuncture also has the capacity to restore mental and emotional balance.

Currently, acupuncture is covered under a naturopathic physician's license only in Connecticut and Arizona. Some naturopathic physicians also have a degree in Oriental medicine and can administer acupuncture in addition to other naturopathic treatments.

Chinese Herbs

Chinese herbal medicine relies on a deep understanding of herbs from the perspective of their actions as "simples" (single herbs), as well as their function in combination with other herbs. Instead of focusing on what illnesses a particular herb treats, the Chinese consider the general effects on the body, e.g., does the herb warm the body? Cause sweating? Increase digestive action? Does it tend to increase fluid production? Cause dryness? These are all examples of an herb's "actions."

Once a Chinese medical practitioner has identified a pattern of imbalance in the body, she can identify the herbs that will best address the situation. Rarely are Chinese herbs prescribed as "simples"; instead, they are combined to create a powerful synergistic blend. Formulas include secondary herbs to balance potential side effects of the major herbs in the formula. A combination of herbs to stop a fever, for example, may contain a small amount of warming herb along with the cooling herbs. The single warming herb moderates the strong cooling action of the other herbs, thereby protecting the body from harsh extremes in temperature. Other herbs may amplify the effects of one of the major herbs in a formula. The herbal combinations always aim to restore balance, or physiological equilibrium, in the body.

Tui Na

The Chinese form of body work known as *tui na* is a richly varied therapeutic modality. A *tui na* master may incorporate deep-tissue work, manipulation, stretching, and energy or "meridian" work in a single treatment session. Gifted *tui na* practitioners treat a wide variety of musculoskeletal conditions.

Qi Gong

This branch of Chinese Medicine applies the wisdom of the body's "subtle energies" in conjunction with the universal life energy. *Qi gong* masters expand upon the understanding of the meridian system in the body and teach students to strengthen these energy currents through daily movement and meditation practices.

AYURVEDIC MEDICINE

Some medical historians cite Ayurvedic medicine as the basis of Chinese medicine. The healing wisdom of India, they contend, moved first into Nepal and Tibet, then gradually filtered into China, and eventually into Japan as well.

Like Chinese medicine, Ayurvedic medicine addresses balance in the body. Instead of focusing on five elements, however, Ayurvedic medicine focuses on three: fire (*pitta*), earth (*kapha*), and air (*vatta*). Ayurvedic diagnosis involves evaluating a patient's constitution according to the predominance of one or more of these elements, or *doshas*. In reality, the *doshas* constantly fluctuate in the body, maintaining a dynamic equilibrium from moment to moment. An Ayurvedic practitioner prescribes treatment according to the patient's constitution. In addition, he or she may include treatments to rectify acute imbalances.

A complete Ayurvedic therapeutic program may include diet, exercise, herbs, meditation, breathing, and physical therapy recommendations. The physical therapies encompass a broad range of treatments, including massage, sound and color therapy, and detoxification techniques.

INDIGENOUS MEDICINE

Indigenous Earth-based cultures the world over possess a profound knowledge of healing. One Chippewa (Ashnabe) teacher described three types of healers in his culture: those who heal with their hands, those who heal with herbs, and those who heal with their minds, through teaching. His path was the last one, although he also had an impressive knowledge of herbs. When a woman approached him for information about a particular plant and its healing properties, he gave her a mystified look. "You're a two-legged, just like me," he said. "Why don't you go ask the plant?"

Many Western scientists assume that indigenous peoples developed their healing methods strictly through trial and error. In reality, most indigenous cultures employ a higher form of investigative science. They know the plants and animals in their locale as intimately as they do their own children. They watch ailing animals to see what they do to heal themselves. Through dreams, they are guided to new plant allies. In quiet moments, they are inspired to use therapies involving minerals, water, air, and fire. Most indigenous peoples have perfected the art of "deep listening," stilling the mind's chatter enough to make room for the quieter, subtler voices of the Earth's inhabitants. This ability to listen deeply has developed healers and therapeutic techniques that sometimes defy scientific explanation.

Many indigenous healers know, for example, that a plant acts more powerfully when one gives thanks and honors its spirit. Distractedly throwing mint in a teapot and brewing an after-dinner tea has a less potent effect than skillfully growing the herb, gathering it with prayer, offering thanks to the Creator, and invoking the healing capacities of that plant ally. This attitude of reverence evokes a different response, a deeper resonance, and a profound opportunity for healing. One's relationship to a plant or element greatly affects its healing power. Western technology has no means of measuring, and thereby justifying, such qualitative differences in administering a healing method.

Native cultures have a deep understanding of "right relationship" with all life forms. Right relationship begins with self and Creator, and circles outward to include one's family, community, and world. "Community" includes all aspects of creation, and relating rightly within that community also includes considering the generations yet to come.

Most indigenous cultures strengthen this weave of Creator, self, community, and world through *ceremony*. Each indigenous culture develops a ceremonial cycle that reflects its relationship with the land and the seasons. If a people must migrate because of famine or invasion, they retain their essence as a culture while adopting the ceremonial cycle of their new home. Ceremonies are specific to different parts of the Earth. Cacti grow well in the desert but not in the rain forest; similarly, ceremonies of the Eastern woodlands do not necessarily make sense in the Southwestern pueblos, even though the indigenous peoples share compatible spiritual concepts.

Ceremony can be a powerful healing tool, encouraging people to reconnect with themselves and their communities. Ceremonies mark individual life transitions as well as the revolving wheel of the seasons. Prayer and ritual can invoke profound healings. Through ceremony we are rooted in place and time, which allows us to expand outward to greet and honor the larger circle of life.

Chapter Three
Home Remedies

The body is wise in its response to changes in the internal and external environment. Symptoms we may regard as nuisances may be the body's way of trying to restore balance in a system that is off-kilter. The home remedies mentioned in this section are meant to stimulate the body's ability to restore balance, rather than merely eradicate symptoms.

Keep in mind that treatments must be individualized to address the needs of a particular person. The following suggestions are not intended as one-size-fits-all prescriptions, but as general guidelines to approaching an acute illness or accident. Please incorporate the suggestions in concert with your own intuition and, when necessary, with the guidance of a physician. (Most of the sections below contain information on "When to consult a physician.")

Once the body's equilibrium is disturbed, whether by overwork, emotional upset, or physical injury, the body will attempt to restore balance. The body's most common response to a disturbance is to generate an inflammatory reaction. Fever, for instance, is an inflammatory response to an overgrowth of a bacteria or virus. The body, in its wisdom, knows that bacteria and viruses can survive only in a very narrow temperature range. Elevating the core body temperature by as little as one or two degrees can make the body completely inhospitable to the invading organisms. Clinical studies show that even virulent spirochetes like syphilis cannot endure temperatures above 106°F. Fever therapy, in this case, would entail slowly elevating, maintaining, and then reducing the body temperature over several hours in a clinical setting. Generally the therapeutic range for a fever is 99–102°F. Please refer to the section of this chapter on "Fevers" for more information on how to work with fevers to restore health.

When a virus takes hold, we say we have "caught a cold." In reality, we are surrounded by viruses and bacteria all the time. As one friend, a devoted bus rider, says, "Riding a public bus in winter is like riding in a petri dish." The bus is a concentrated microcosm of the larger environment. In truth, the Earth as a whole is a "petri dish" teeming with microorganisms that are both harmful and beneficial to human life.

At least two major factors determine whether or not someone "comes down with a cold" or other illness while riding in the "petri dish." One is the strength of the virus. Some pathogens are more virulent than others. The second factor is the strength of the human being (or, more precisely, the condition of the human being's immune system). Someone who eats well, enjoys work, has a loving family environment, and exercises regularly will probably be less susceptible to a virus than someone who eats fast food, works thirteen hours a day, sleeps four hours a night, hates his or her job, and argues incessantly with her mate.

What are the basic principles that support health? Four major areas contribute to overall health and well-being:

- nutrition
- exercise
- mental/emotional health
- trust in and connection with "divinity," i.e., a supportive force larger than oneself

All these factors function synergistically to strengthen health. Restoring health may involve addressing one or more of these factors. Making changes in one area almost certainly will bring about changes in another area. One friend notes that her tendency to overeat diminishes when she meditates twenty minutes before going to sleep at night (mind/spirit affecting body). I notice that I am calmer and more patient when I exercise aerobically at least twenty minutes per day (body affecting mind/spirit).

The newly emerging field of psychoneuroimmunology explores this interconnectedness of mind and body, which occurs through the actions of the endocrine, nervous, and immune systems. As westerners, we are learning what easterners and indigenous peoples have known for thousands of years: we are "webbed," interconnected within ourselves and with the larger pattern of Creation on this planet. The content of our minds affects our bodies, just as surely as our physical state affects our mental and emotional well-being.

The best home care is preventive care. Investing in good food, in time for exercise and relaxation, and in loving communication with friends and family will repay you many times over. The suggestions that follow are meant to support you when, despite your best efforts, you are unable to maintain health. Ideally, these treatments will help speed the healing process and quicken the return from inflammation to optimal health (see Chapter 1, "Paradigm of Health and Disease"). The aim is to support, not suppress, the body's attempts to heal.

Agatha Thrash, M.D. and Calvin Thrash, M.D. have devoted their lives to administering natural therapeutics for a wide range of illnesses. Their book, *Home Remedies*, is packed with wisdom and therapeutic suggestions. They remind readers that

> the natural remedies require time to apply and a simple skill
> that demands carefulness more than expertise. Because few

are willing to give the time and care, the natural remedies are dying out from among us. It is not that natural remedies are less effective than drug remedies, but drug administration makes personal nursing care much less necessary. Simple remedies are not as dramatic, but are generally more effective, and they have far fewer side effects.

ACNE

Skin eruptions can be painful, irritating, and embarrassing. Recalling Chapter 1's "Laws of Cure," skin irritations and eruptions are less serious than internal-organ diseases because they are closer to the surface of the body. (Try telling that to a teenager getting ready for the prom!) Treating acne requires persistence and a willingness to make lifestyle changes.

Nutritional therapy: From a Chinese perspective, an accumulation of dampness and heat causes acne. Foods that increase dampness in the body include cold foods (ice cream and iced drinks), raw foods, fatty foods (nuts, corn chips, fatty meats, cheese), and sweets. Foods that cause heat accumulation include meat (chicken is the most warming), seafood, and spicy foods.

Generally, include more whole grains, fruits, and vegetables in the diet. These foods are high in fiber and help stimulate elimination of toxins from the body. When the digestive system is overburdened and cannot discharge waste, the body pushes out waste products through the skin.

Eat foods that support the liver. Skin health is intimately linked with the liver, which is responsible for removal of many toxins from the body. Liver-supporting foods include beets (root and greens), olive oil, garlic, and lemon juice. Drink plenty of filtered water, at least two to three quarts per day. Water flushes toxins from the body and moisturizes the skin.

Nutritional supplements:

- Vitamin A reduces sebum secretion from the oil glands and encourages tissue healing. This vitamin must be taken at high doses for at least three months to produce an effect. Unfortunately, high doses of vitamin A have potentially toxic side effects. Signs of toxicity include headache, fatigue, constipation, dry or scaly skin, mouth fissures, brittle nails, hair loss, nausea, and vomiting. Vitamin A therapy should be followed by liver screening tests.

   NOTE: Consult a physician before beginning vitamin A therapy.

- Beta carotene is the precursor to vitamin A and can be taken at high doses (up to 150,000 IU) without risk of side effects. Unfortunately, beta carotene does not have the effect of reducing sebum production but will encourage healing of skin tissue.

- Vitamin E also encourages skin healing and acts as an antioxidant, preventing lipid oxidation and cell damage. Take 400 IU per day.

- Zinc stimulates immune function, promotes skin healing, and acts as an antioxidant. Take 30–60 mg per day.

- Vitamin C has many functions, chief among them being antioxidant activity and connective-tissue healing. Only three mammals—guinea pigs, primates, and humans—do not produce their own vitamin C internally and must rely on their food supply to obtain it. Most humans need far more than the 40 mg of vitamin C that is listed as the Recommended Daily Allowance. For acne treatment, take at least one gram of vitamin C three times per day. Gradually build up to taking nine grams of vitamin C (three grams, three times per day). The body begins to use up more C if a steady supply is available. You cannot take too much—

any unused amount of this water-soluble vitamin is passed in the urine.

CAUTION: if you have a history of kidney stones, be sure to drink plenty of water with vitamin C therapy, at least two to three quarts of filtered water per day. Whether or not you have kidney stones, use buffered vitamin C preparations. Never suddenly discontinue Vitamin C supplementation. Instead, gradually reduce your dosage over at least two weeks.

Physical therapies:

- Avoid harsh soaps and ointments that contain sulfur. These cause excessive drying and can irritate the skin.
- Wash the face at least twice per day with a washcloth to stimulate the removal of dead skin.
- Alternate hot and cold applications to the face to stimulate circulation and encourage healing (see Chapter 2, "Hydrotherapy" section). Add *Calendula succus* (fresh plant extract) to the cold-water application.
- Avoid picking at the pimples and blackheads. Squeezing and picking can cause scarring and further tissue irritation.

Botanical medicines: The following herbal tea encourages liver health and skin healing. Drink 3–4 cups of herbal tea per day, or two dropperfuls of tincture four times per day.

Combine:

> dandelion root (*Taraxacum officinalis*)—2 parts, by weight
> yellow dock (*Rumex crispus*)—1 part
> red clover blossoms (*Trifolium pratens*)—1 part
> Oregon grape root (*Berberis aquafolium*)—1 part
> nettles (*Urtica urens*)—1 part
> licorice (*Glycerrhiza glabra*)—1/2 part

Homeopathic remedies: Consult with a homeopathic practitioner to determine the best remedy for you. Generally, a constitutional remedy is more helpful than a prescription based on acute acne symptoms.

When to consult a physician:
- If acne persists, despite following the preceding therapeutic guidelines for at least three months.
- If acne scars the face.
- If acne appears after adolescence, or persists after twenty years of age.

ALLERGIC REACTIONS, HAY FEVER

Hay fever is a relatively mild, although very uncomfortable, form of allergic reaction. Treatment of hay fever should begin at least half a year before the onset of allergy season. Supportive therapies may include dietary changes, nutritional supplements, herbal preparations, and stress reduction so that the body's immune system is in optimal condition when hay-fever season arrives.

Mild to moderate allergic reactions may manifest in a variety of ways, from minor headaches or digestive disturbances, to itchy, blotchy skin rashes. Severe allergic reactions, called "anaphylactic shock," cause swelling of the airways. Sufferers often gasp and wheeze, trying to get air through the swollen passageways. In very severe cases, the airway can become completely blocked, causing respiratory arrest.

The following suggestions are for hay fever and mild to moderate allergic reactions:
- Nettles, in freeze-dried capsules, two capsules every two hours. In freeze-dried form, nettles have been shown to benefit 50 percent of patients suffering with hay-fever symptoms.
- Eliminate food and inhalant sensitivities, if known.

- For hay-fever symptoms, reduce or eliminate foods that encourage mucus formation, e.g., dairy products, sugar, and alcohol.

Homeopathic remedies: 30c potency, to be taken every 30–60 minutes during an acute attack, or twice per day during an ongoing allergy reaction. Stop the remedy once you notice signs of improvement.

- *Apis*—edema, swelling, and blotching of the skin.
- *Carbo veg*—"air hunger," wants to be fanned.
- *Arsenicum*—allergic reaction to food; vomiting and diarrhea, burning pains, wants small sips of warm water.

BOILS

A boil is caused by a staphylococcus infection localized in a hair follicle. The body's immune system attempts to contain the infection by "walling off" the infected area, leading to increased pressure and pain. Often a boil will cause sharp, even excruciating pain before it comes to a head and releases its pus and blood. The suggestions below are intended to abort the boil, if caught in its early stages, or to speed the resolution and healing of a ripening boil.

- The skin is the largest organ of elimination in the body. When other elimination systems (chiefly the liver, colon, bladder, and lungs) become overburdened, the body will throw off waste products through the skin. Boils often occur when someone is tired and run down; the immune system is overburdened, and the organs of elimination cannot process wastes properly. Encourage elimination by increasing water intake to at least two quarts per day. Eat more whole grains, steamed vegetables, and other fiber-rich foods that will encourage elimination through the colon rather than the skin.

- From a Chinese medical perspective, boils are caused by an accumulation of dampness and heat in the body. Boils are more common in hot, damp climates and occur more frequently during hot, humid summers. When boils begin to form, avoid foods and activities that will increase dampness and heat. Dampness-forming foods include sugar, dairy products (especially ice cream), and greasy foods. Heating foods include alcohol, meat, and hot spices. Living in a damp basement or a damp climate can increase dampness in the body. Saunas, sweat lodges, and steam baths can increase heat in the body.

Homeopathic remedies: 30c potency. Take the remedy 3–4 times per day until the pain and swelling resolve (early stages), or until the boil erupts and discharges (later stage).

- *Belladonna*—early stage, when the area is red, swollen, and painful.
- *Hepar sulph*—for later stage, when the boil begins to develop a pocket of pus. *Hepar sulph* will cause the boil to discharge or resolve.
- *Silica*—will encourage the boil to discharge. *Silica* also can speed the healing of a boil that is slow to resolve after discharge.

Hydrotherapy: you can increase circulation to the affected area, thus encouraging the boil to come to a head, by alternating hot and cold wet towels to the area. Cover the area with a hot wet towel for five minutes, followed by a cold wet towel for one minute. Alternate the towels at least three times. Always end with a cold application. Repeat the treatment in the morning and evening. The hot towels will increase circulation and soften the skin to encourage discharge from the boil. To avoid spreading the infection, be sure to wash the towels after each treatment. Do not share towels with any household members during the time you are treating the boil.

When to consult a physician:

- If a boil develops near the eyes or nose—the infection can spread to the brain via the facial artery.
- If the boil does not resolve within 4–5 days.
- If the boil erupts but does not heal.

BROKEN BONES

Broken bones are serious injuries that require medical attention. Get to your primary-care physician or to a hospital as soon as possible. The following suggestions are meant for emergency first aid, to decrease the trauma of a bone break. Also included are home-care suggestions to speed bone healing.

- Protect the area of the bone break. For a compound fracture (where the broken bone has penetrated the skin), cover the area with a clean, soft cloth. Seek appropriate medical attention.
- Immobilize the area. Further movement of a broken bone, especially of a compound fracture, can increase damage to surrounding soft tissue.
- Research in the early twentieth century demonstrated that bones heal more quickly if they are bandaged and allowed to move, rather than being immobilized in a cast, because the stress of movement and weight-bearing stimulates healing in the bone. Although you may not be able to convince your physician to eliminate the cast, you can move the limb as much as possible within the constraints of the cast and request a walking cast for a broken fibula or tibia (lower leg).

Homeopathic remedies: 30c potency

- *Arnica*—for acute pain, swelling, trauma to bone and soft tissues. Take one dose every 15–30 minutes as needed for the first 3–4 hours after injury. Continue taking Arnica as needed for the first 36–48 hours after injury.

- *Eupatorium*—specific for bone pain. Begin taking after acute swelling and trauma have passed.
- *Symphytum*—stimulates bone healing.
- *Calcarea phosphorica*—helps reduce bone pain. *Calc phos* is also available as a cell salt, usually in 6x potency.
- *Hypericum*—for shooting, nerve-like pain
- *Ruta*—stimulates healing of the periosteum (surface layer of the bone). *Ruta* will encourage the final stages of healing, e.g., resolve pain that persists after a cast is removed.

Hydrotherapy can increase circulation and encourage healing. Apply alternating hot (five minutes) and cold (one minute) wet towels to the limb *opposite* the one that is broken. Increasing circulation in one limb reflexively increases circulation in the opposite limb. This method is especially helpful if the limb is bandaged or in a cast.

NOTE: Never apply heat or cold to a cast or splint.

BRUISES

Cayenne liniment: add one tablespoon cayenne pepper to one cup apple-cider vinegar. Allow to sit for a week. Apply the liniment to bruised areas to increase circulation.

CAUTION: Apply to unbroken skin only. Avoid contact with the eyes.

Homeopathic remedies: 30c potency
- *Arnica*—is the principle remedy, especially for injuries to the head. Take every 30–60 minutes immediately following injury, then 2–3 times per day until you note improvement. Taking *Arnica* immediately after an injury may stop bruising and swelling completely.

- *Hypericum*—injuries to highly enervated areas (e.g., eyeball, hands, feet, genitals) or in case of nerve damage or bruising.
- *Aconite*—hot, throbbing, no discoloration; patient is anxious.
- *Belladonna*—discolored, throbbing, hot.

Hydrotherapy: alternating hot and cold applications to increase blood circulation.

When to consult a physician:
- If you see red streaks developing around the bruise (usually moving from the site of injury toward the heart), a sign of possible infection.
- If the area continues to swell.
- If a bruise persists for more than 7–10 days.
- If you bruise frequently and easily (a possible sign of bioflavonoid deficiency, clotting disorder, diabetes, or other condition).

BURNS

Minor burns respond well to home treatment. The sooner you treat the burn, the less damage will occur and the quicker the healing will take place.

CAUTION: Do not apply butter or any kind of oil-based cream to the burn. Putting fat or oil on a burn is like throwing fat on a fire—it will intensify the effect of the burn.

Hydrotherapy: Immerse the burned area in cold water as soon as possible.

Homeopathic remedies: 30c potencies. Repeat one dose (three pellets) of the remedy every 2–3 hours until pain and inflammation diminishes, then stop the remedy.

First-degree burn (pain, inflammation, redness)
- *Cantharis*—for burning pain that improves with cold applications. Also for second-degree burn with blister formation.

- *Hypericum*—for extremely tender, painful burns; shooting, nerve-like pain.
- *Apis*—for stinging, itching pain.

Second-degree burn (inflammation, redness and blistering of the skin)
- *Cantharis*—for burning pain that improves with cold applications.

Third-degree burn (charring of the skin, tissue damage)
- *Cantharis*—for burning pain that improves with cold applications. Blister formation.
- *Causticum*—for severe burns, including chemical burns.

Botanical treatments:
- *Aloe vera*—soothes burns and encourages healing. The best, and cheapest, source is fresh leaves from the aloe plant. Open the leaves and use the gel-like substance inside. (The skin of the aloe leaf is not effective for treating burns.) The second best source is bottled aloe vera, available in health food stores. Look for a product without preservatives. Beware of oil-based creams and lotions, which will worsen the effects of the burn.
- *Hypericum* (St. John's Wort)—encourages healing of burns. Use crushed fresh blossoms in a poultice. You also can apply diluted Hypericum tincture to the burn. (Dilute one part of the tincture in ten parts water.) Hypericum oil may be used to *prevent* burns if applied hourly to the skin during sun exposure. For sun-sensitive, fair-skinned people, use Hypericum oil as an emergency back-up only. Hypericum is not as strong as a sunblock, but can be helpful if you are stranded somewhere without any other form of protection.

  CAUTION: Do not use oil of Hypericum *on* burns.

When to consult a physician:

- If you have a second- or third-degree burn (blistering and/ or charring of the skin).
- If the burn becomes infected.
- If pain and swelling associated with the burn has not resolved within 4–5 days. (The actual burn, especially with blistering, may take longer to heal, but the pain should stop within 1–2 days.)
- If the burn covers more than 10–15 percent of the body.

COLDS

A cold is a healing reaction, the body attempting to regain balance after having been affected by physical or emotional stresses. Fever and mucus discharges are a way of ridding the body of external pernicious influences (such as wind, cold, and heat—see Chapter 2's section on "Chinese Medicine") and built-up waste. Colds do not require treatment; they *are* the treatment. You can speed up the healing process, however, by encouraging the body to discharge the disturbance and return to optimal health (see Chapter 1, "Paradigm of Health and Disease").

How To Catch a Cold

Go to a relative's house for Thanksgiving. Eat everything in sight, until you are well beyond pleasantly full. Get into an argument with the brother you haven't seen for three years. Relive every childhood pattern you thought you had outgrown. Stand in the doorway, saying goodbye, without buttoning your coat, for at least twenty minutes. Get in the car, drive home, and watch football on TV. When dinner time arrives, eat more even though you're not hungry. (Besides, you deserve something delicious because your team lost again in the Kumquat Bowl.)

General recommendations for a cold:

- Rest! Get in bed as soon as possible, and continue to rest for at least twenty-four hours after the symptoms resolve.

- Stop eating for at least one full day, and drink plenty of fluids. Digesting food requires energy that the body might better utilize fighting a viral or bacterial overgrowth. Increasing fluids will thin mucus, making it easier to expel. Fluids also will help prevent dehydration if you have a fever.

- Wet-socks treatment (see Chapter 2, "Hydrotherapy" section) before going to sleep. Begin the treatment with the very first symptoms, and you may completely abort the cold. Continue the treatment every night until the symptoms resolve.

- Encourage sweating to push out what the Chinese call "external pernicious influences" (EPIs), such as an invasion of wind, heat, or cold. Simmer a tablespoon of fresh ginger in two cups of water for ten minutes, or steep a tablespoon of yarrow blossom tea in two cups boiling water for ten minutes. Draw a hot bath. Sip the tea while relaxing in the bath. Once you begin to sweat, get out of the bath, towel dry, and get into bed. Wrap up in warm blankets and allow yourself to sweat. Make sure that you are not exposed to drafts or chills during this treatment. Your pores are open, and therefore more susceptible to drafts and chills. In the morning, take a shower to rinse off the sweat and excreted toxins.

  CAUTION: Sweating therapy can further weaken someone who is debilitated (elderly persons, or those with long-term chronic illnesses). Also, children often do not need such aggressive therapy.

- *Yin qiao san*—a Chinese patent medicine for "wind heat invasion." Symptoms include sore throat, feeling more feverish than chilled, slight headache, and yellowish mucus discharge. Do not take the remedy if you feel more chills than fever and have no sore throat—the formula is very cooling. *Yin qiao san* is meant to cause sweating to help push out wind and heat. Make sure to avoid drafts and chills after taking the remedy. Take three tablets four times per day for sore throat. If you have a fever, increase the dosage to three tablets every 2–3 hours. This remedy is for the very beginning of a cold, within twenty-four hours (optimally, within 1–2 hours) of the onset of symptoms.

- Salt-water gargle—excellent for sore throats. Salt water soothes the throat and kills bacteria and viruses. Add two teaspoons of sea salt (better than mined table salt) per glass of warm water.

- Hold Echinacea and/or Goldenseal tincture (one dropperful) at the back of the throat as long as possible, then swallow. This is only for the brave! These herbs are strong and have a local antimicrobial effect on the sore throat, as well as working internally on the cold or flu. Repeat every 3–4 hours, as needed.

- Take Hydrastis (Goldenseal) and Echinacea tincture or capsules. These herbs will boost the immune system when taken internally. Take two dropperfuls of tincture or two capsules every 2–4 hours, depending on the severity of the cold.

  —*Six years old:* half the adult dosage (one dropperful every 2–4 hours)

  —*Three years old:* one-quarter the adult dosage

  —*One year old:* one-sixth the adult dosage

  Hydrastis has a drying effect on the mucous membranes, making it ideal for any kind of upper-respiratory infection (sinus, lung, nasal). Echinacea stimulates white blood cell production and activity.

  NOTE: Some people are sensitive to Hydrastis (Goldenseal). If you notice a skin rash or other allergic reaction developing, stop taking Goldenseal.

- Herbal teas also can help speed the resolution of a cold.

Combine equal parts:

| yarrow | blue vervain |
| mint | ginger (dried or fresh) |

This is a warming tea and may cause sweating. Add one tablespoon of the above mix to one cup boiling water and steep for ten minutes. Drink one cup 3–4 times per day.

Homeopathic remedies: 30c potency. Take three pellets 2–3 times per day until improvement is noted, then stop taking the remedy.

- *Occilococcinum*—use at the very first hint of a cold, right after the first sneeze. The remedy will not be effective after the first twenty-four hours. Take six of the small pellets every 3–4 hours. You do not need to take the entire tube, as the directions on the bottle may suggest— that is a way of selling you more tubes! Remember that homeopathic remedies act according to frequency of dosage, not the amount.

- *Aconite*—take after the first sneeze, when feeling anxious or fretful; symptoms may have developed following exposure to a cold, dry wind.

- *Allium cepa*—lots of mucus drainage, sore upper lip, excoriating discharge from the nose, bland discharge from eyes; feels worse in a warm room, better in fresh air.

- *Arsenicum*—affected by changes in weather; thin, painful, burning discharges; patient seeks warmth.

- *Pulsatilla*—thick, bland discharges, often green or yellow. Changing symptoms: pains move around and do not localize. Patient feels better outside, worse in stuffy room. Wants company, wants to be held (children), improves with sympathy. Best for late-stage, "ripe" colds.

- *Gelsemium*—slow onset, for colds that begin in warm weather or during a mild winter. Patient feels achy, the limbs heavy, as in a Southern swamp in August. No thirst.

- *Bryonia*—feels worse with motion, better with pressure. Very hot, very dry, aches all over. Great thirst for cold drinks.
- *Nux vomica*—very chilly, even while bundled up in bed. Worsens with slight uncovering, or the least movement. Feels chilled from drinking. Aching in limbs and back. Nose stuffed at night. May have upset stomach or other digestive symptoms.

When to consult a physician:
- If you have followed the above suggestions (especially regarding rest) and still have symptoms after seven days.
- If a child has a severe sore throat—especially if she is drooling profusely and cannot swallow.
- If a child has cold and fever symptoms accompanied by a stiff neck or arched back.
- If sore-throat symptoms persist longer than three days.
- If you have a fever above 102°F that does not respond to the suggestions in the "Fever" section of this chapter.

COLIC

Be sure to rule out any possible organic causes of colic, such as bowel obstruction or lactose intolerance. Any major problems usually become apparent from a couple of days to a week after birth.

Nutritional therapy:
- Breast-feed children as long as possible. Developing infant digestive and immune systems are not able to handle solid foods until at least six months of age. Many children develop food intolerances because of early exposure to food other than human breast milk. Recent research links adult-onset diabetes with early exposure to cow's milk.
- Smaller, more frequent feedings.

- Skin-to-skin contact can soothe and calm the infant, helping the digestive system to function more smoothly.
- Breast-feeding mothers may experiment with eliminating certain foods to discover any foods that are irritating the infant. Cabbage, caffeine, onions, garlic, and highly spiced foods are common irritants. Laxatives, such as large amounts of prune juice (more than one cup per day), also may irritate the baby's digestive system.
- Feed your baby in a quiet, relaxed environment whenever possible.
- Slippery elm is a good food substitute for extreme cases of colic, acting as a demulcent to soothe the infant's digestive tract. Mix two tablespoons of slippery-elm-bark powder with a small amount of sweetener (maple syrup or molasses). Add hot water or hot milk—mother's milk, if you are still breast feeding—until the mixture is the consistency of porridge. Feed the baby slippery elm in place of other solid foods.

Botanical medicines:

- For breast-feeding mothers, drink chamomile tea to soothe the infant's digestive system.
- For children receiving formula, add 1/4 cup chamomile tea to a bottle of formula.
- Aromatic seeds have a soothing effect on the digestive system. Prepare an infusion of one of the following seeds (one teaspoon of seed per cup of water): cardamom, fennel, anise, cumin. Strain and add 1/4 cup to infant's formula, or drink a cup of this tea 10–15 minutes before breast feeding.

Physical therapy:

Gently massage the infant's abdomen with a good vegetable oil (e.g., sesame, almond, or other cold-pressed oil) in a clockwise, circular motion.

Homeopathic remedies: 30c potency

- *Magnesium phosphorica*—cramping pain that improves with warm applications.
- *Chamomilla*—child is extremely irritable, wants to be carried, then demands to be put down. Inconsolable. One cheek is red, the other pale.
- *Cholocynthis*—cramping, abdominal pain that is relieved by pressure and by drawing the knees toward the chest.
- *Bryonia*—feels worse following the slightest motion; generally irritable.

When to consult a physician:

- If the infant is losing weight.
- If colic routinely disturbs the infant's sleep cycle.

CONSTIPATION

A healthy person with a healthy digestive tract will have one to three bowel movements per day. Normal stools are light brown with no mucus or blood, well-formed, soft, and easy to pass.

Persons suffering with constipation go two or three days without having a bowel movement. Difficulty passing stools does not necessarily mean one is constipated. The following suggestions will also benefit patients who have daily bowel movements that are difficult to pass.

- Stop taking laxatives. If laxatives are used over a long period of time, the bowel loses its ability to stimulate movement (peristalsis) in the colon. Eventually, the body grows resistant to the laxatives, and movement in the colon ceases altogether. During the bowel-retraining time, you may use herbal laxatives 2–3 times per week, before going to sleep, to replace the action of other laxatives. Decrease the herbs by half a dose per week until you no longer need laxatives to stimulate bowel activity.

- Increase water consumption to at least two quarts per day. Often constipation results from simple lack of fluid in the digestive tract.

- Eliminate coffee, black tea, and other stimulants. Coffee has the effect of increasing gut peristalsis (the contraction of smooth muscle in the digestive tract), but also acts as a diuretic, decreasing fluid in the body. (Each cup of coffee results in the loss of two cups of fluid from the body.) Water and herbal teas are better sources of fluid.

- Increase fiber in the diet. Fiber creates bulk in the intestines, which helps stimulate elimination. The simplest way to increase fiber is to eat foods as close as possible to their natural state. Brown rice, for example, contains more fiber than white rice, which contains more fiber than white-rice flour. Apples have more fiber than apple juice. Focus on whole grains, steamed vegetables, and fresh fruits in the diet.

- Develop a regular rhythm for elimination. Some people become constipated because they never make time to have a bowel movement. Generally, early morning is the best time to set aside for bowel training. (From a Chinese perspective, each organ has a time of day when it is most active; large intestine time is 5–7 a.m.) Drink a glass of warm water or herb tea when you get out of bed. Fifteen minutes later, sit on the toilet for at least five minutes. Do not strain or try to force a bowel movement. Get up after five minutes and go about your day. Avoid reading or doing any other activity while sitting on the toilet, to ensure that the mind and body associate the toilet with elimination only. Over time, the body will get used to the rhythm and respond with regular bowel movements.

- Never repress an urge to defecate.

- Exercise at least twenty minutes per day, three days per week (the minimum amount of exercise to maintain aerobic fitness). Exercise stimulates colon activity.

Homeopathic remedies: 30c potency

- *Nux vomica*—"ineffectual urging to stool," never feel completely emptied. Overuse of laxatives. Chilly, irritable.
- *Sulphur*—frequent urge with incomplete evacuation. Hard, dry, black stools expelled with great effort, pain, and burning, especially around the anus. Alternating constipation and diarrhea. 5 a.m. diarrhea.
- *Bryonia*—dry mouth, dry lips, dry tongue. Stools dry and hard, as if burnt. Thirst for large quantities of water.
- *Calc carb*—feels better the longer the patient doesn't have a bowel movement.

Botanical remedies:

- *Psyllium seeds*—one or two tablespoons taken with water or diluted fruit juice after each meal increases bulk in the stool. The seeds are also mucilaginous, helping to lubricate the stool. With any bulk stool softener, you must increase water intake; otherwise, the fiber will bind the stool and make the constipation even worse.
- *Aloe vera*—aloe vera gel, made from the inner part of the leaves, is a mild laxative that also helps to lubricate stools. Take one tablespoon after each meal. The skin of the aloe vera leaf is a powerful cathartic that should be used only in extreme situations, not on a regular basis.
- *Buckthorn (Cascara sagrada)*—stimulates peristalsis. Some people experience intestinal cramping with cascara. With long-term use, cascara can have the same side effects as chemical laxatives, so short-term usage (1–2 months maximum) is best during the bowel retraining program.
- *Cassia senna*—similar to cascara in its actions and effects.
- *Slippery elm (Ulmus fulva)*—helps to lubricate the stool and increase bulk.
- *Smooth Move* (made by Traditional Medicinals)—a good prepared tea that combines several of the above herbs. As noted above, some people experience intestinal cramping after taking cascara.

When to consult a physician:

- If more than a week passes without having a bowel movement.
- If you follow the above suggestions and still experience constipation. Your physician can test for other causes.

COUGHS

Steam inhalation: three to five drops of peppermint oil added to a pan of boiling water. Drape a towel over your head and inhale the steam for 5–10 minutes, or until the vapor begins to cool. Peppermint oil has high concentrations of free menthol, soothing irritated mucous-membrane tissues (which constitute the lining of the entire respiratory tract). Menthol also helps to fight viral and bacterial infections. A steam inhalation at the earliest signs of a cold or flu may abort an illness before it starts.

Essential oils (applied to the chest and neck)

- Combine ten drops each of thyme, rosemary, eucalyptus, and camphorated oil. Rub ten drops of this mixture on the chest and neck 2–3 times per day. Stop if the skin develops a rash or becomes excessively irritated. Some reddening of the skin is normal, as the oils will draw circulation into the area.
- Olbas oil, a commercial preparation, also can be used following the directions given above.

CUTS

- Apply direct pressure to the wound, pressing the area with a clean cloth, bandanna, or T-shirt until bleeding stops.
- Wash the wound with water, or soap and water if available. Washing a puncture wound is especially important, as bacteria can move into a deep wound and remain after the area has healed on the skin surface. Even such virulent

bacterial infections as tetanus and rabies can be aborted by carefully washing the wound. Of course, you cannot rely on soap and water alone.

- Apply *Calendula succus* (fresh plant extract of calendula). If stinging results, dilute one part *Calendula succus* in ten parts water. The mixture may be stored in a sterilized spray bottle for use as an anti-bacterial spray. If soap and water are unavailable, applying *Calendula succus* can take the place of washing.

- *Yunnan pai yao* is a Chinese herbal formula that was brought to the West from Vietnam, where U.S. soldiers witnessed its seemingly miraculous effects. The powder can be packed into wounds to stop bleeding, or taken internally. *Each package comes with one small red pill, which is to be used only for severe hemorrhaging.* The orange-powder capsules, however, may be taken internally, one pill 3–4 times per day, to stop bleeding. Stop taking the medicine as soon as the bleeding stops.

Homeopathic remedies: 30c potency. Take three pellets every 15–30 minutes for acute bleeding. Stop taking the remedy when the bleeding stops.

- *Arnica*—helps stop bleeding, especially bleeding associated with soft-tissue injury.
- *Phosphorous*—for arterial bleeding (bright red blood, usually cascading in spurts).
- *Belladonna*—helps infection, especially staph and strep.
- *Mag phos*—releases muscle tension associated with cuts and other physical trauma.
- *Ferrum phos*—helps stop bleeding.

When to consult a physician:

- If you are bitten by an animal (wild or domesticated).
- If you cannot completely clean a cut or wound. ("Dirty" wounds, especially puncture wounds, may develop tetanus.)

- If you cannot stop the bleeding with direct pressure.
- If infection develops during healing.

DIAPER RASH

Most diaper rashes are caused by prolonged exposure to wet, soiled diapers. Keeping the infant's bottom as dry as possible decreases the chances of developing diaper rash.

General recommendations:
- Change diapers frequently, right after each bowel movement.
- Expose baby's bottom to light and air as often as possible.
- Use cotton diapers without plastic pants whenever possible; cotton breathes more than plastic-coated diapers. Use wool "soakers" instead of plastic pants.
- For severe rashes, apply calendula ointment and/or dust with calendula powder. Calendula promotes skin healing and has antibacterial action.
- Use arrowroot powder or bentonite clay instead of commercial baby powders.
- Use olive oil instead of Vaseline or commercial ointments, which have chemical additives that may irritate the baby's skin.
- Wash diapers with soap flakes. Avoid harsh detergents. Add vinegar to the final rinse water, and dry diapers in the sunshine if possible.

For severe rashes:
- Apply comfrey-root ointment to the diaper rash. Comfrey leaf does not contain as much allantoin, the active constituent that promotes skin healing.
- Apply Calendula ointment, which also promotes skin healing.
- Avoid ointments with goldenseal, as this herb may irritate sensitive tissue in the genital area.

When to consult a physician:
- If you have tried the above suggestions and the rash has persisted for more than a week.
- If the skin is raw or bleeding

DIARRHEA

General recommendations:
- Fast or reduce food intake until the diarrhea has passed.
- Increase water intake to avoid dehydration, especially in young children. For adults, drink at least two to three liters of fluid (dilute juices—half water, half juice) each day.
- Dissolve one tablespoon of bentonite clay in a glass of water and drink the clay solution. The clay will draw irritants and toxins from the intestines.
- Eat burnt toast (one or two slices), or activated charcoal dissolved in water. Dissolve one tablespoon of the charcoal in a glass of water and drink. The carbon will absorb toxins and reduce fluid loss.
  NOTE: Activated charcoal will turn the stool black.
- Slippery-elm-bark gruel is easy to digest and soothes the digestive tract. Combine 1/4 cup powdered slippery elm with 3/4 cup water. Bring to a boil, then simmer for approximately five minutes. You also can add one or two tablespoons of slippery elm to oatmeal or other cooked cereal. Eat several tablespoons of the slippery elm gruel every 2–3 hours.

Homeopathic remedies: 30c potency
- *Arsenicum*—for explosive diarrhea with vomiting. Patient is exhausted, restless, anxious; desires hot drinks, in small sips.
- *Bryonia*—following exposure to cold, dry wind, or after a fright.

- *Chamomilla*—diarrhea with teething (infants); grass-green stools with undigested food. The diarrhea has mucus and blood, and smells like rotten eggs.
- *Cholocynthis*—frequent urging, severe colicky pains, relieved by pressure and bending double.
- *Nux vomica*—diarrhea caused by "dietary indiscretion" (eating too much or eating heavy, rich foods). Diarrhea alternating with constipation. Frequent urging, often with no passing of stool; irritable; chilly.
- *Pulsatilla*—diarrhea from rich foods and pastries. Diarrhea at night. Diarrhea from taking cold drinks. Variable—no two stools alike.
- *Sulphur*—diarrhea drives patient out of bed at 5 a.m. Stools are painless, variable in consistency and amount. Red anus.
- *Gelsemium*—Nervous diarrhea ("stage fright").

When to consult a physician:
- If the diarrhea persists for more than two days.
- If a high fever (above 102°F) accompanies the diarrhea
- If you see pus or blood in the diarrhea
- If you have severe, continuous abdominal pain with the diarrhea.

EARACHE

Earaches are especially common in children, in large part because the developing eustachian tubes do not effectively drain the ear. Whether young or old, the pain associated with ear infections is usually intense and requires immediate care.

The best treatment is prevention. Many children respond well to dietary changes. Eliminating dairy and sugar reduces mucus-forming foods; dairy and wheat are the two most common food allergens in North America. Sometimes removing these three foods—milk, sugar, and wheat—is enough to stop recurrent ear infections.

Most children with chronic ear infections are caught on a merry-go-round of antibiotic treatments. The antibiotics clear the infection, but another quickly follows, usually within 4–6 weeks. Antibiotics wipe out the good bacteria in the body, as well as the invading bacteria in the ear. After antibiotic treatment, the body is more susceptible to infection.

Keeping the ears warm and covered when outdoors also helps prevent ear infections, as does increasing vitamin C during the cold season. For children, 500 mg of vitamin C twice per day is an adequate dosage. Adults may supplement 2–3 grams twice per day.

The following suggestions are for acute ear infections, when preventive measures have not succeeded:

General recommendations:

- Sit the patient near a 40-watt light bulb, with the ear close enough to feel warmth, but not close enough to cause burning. Carefully monitor. The warmth will soothe ear pain and increase circulation in the area, which brings more immune cells to fight the infection.

Hydrotherapy:

- Alternate hot and cold applications to the ear. Wring out a washcloth in water as hot as you can stand and apply for five minutes to the ear. Follow with a cold application (a wet washcloth put in the freezer, or a bag of frozen peas) for one minute. Repeat the cycle, alternating hot and cold, at least three times. Always end with a cold application.
- Wet-socks treatment at bedtime (see "Hydrotherapy" section, Chapter 2).
- Constitutional hydrotherapy treatment once per day (see "Hydrotherapy" section, Chapter 2).

Botanical therapy:

- *Oil of mullein and/or garlic*—Place two or three drops of gently warmed oil in the ear. (Warm the oil by placing the bottle in a bowl of hot water for a couple of minutes.) Mullein oil reduces pain and inflammation. Both garlic and mullein have antimicrobial action.

    CAUTION: Use ear drops only if the tympanic membrane (eardrum) is not broken.

- *Echinacea and goldenseal tincture or capsules*—Dose according to age

    —*Twelve and older:* full dose (two dropperfuls, or two capsules every 2–4 hours)

    —*Six years old:* half the adult dosage (one dropperful, or one capsule every 2–4 hours)

    —*Three years old:* one-quarter the adult dosage

    —*One year old:* one-sixth the adult dosage

Homeopathic remedies: 30c potency

- *Aconite*—earache begins after exposure to cold, dry wind. Bright red ears, high fever, sudden onset. Very sensitive to noise. Sharp pain. Anxious, restless. Thirst for cold drinks. Onset after shock.

- *Belladonna*—sudden, violent onset. Dilated pupils. Throbbing blood vessels in the neck. Pain causes delirium. Child may have nightmares and call out in sleep. Throbbing, shooting, sharp pains. No thirst with fever. Red-hot throbbing ear.

- *Chamomilla*—irritable; intense pain. One cheek is red, the other pale. The child wants to be held and carried, yet arches her back. Inconsolable. Earaches from teething. Grass-green stool.

- *Ferrum phos*—first stage of infection, before pus develops. Pulsating, throbbing pain. Flushed face. High fever with few symptoms. Use when Belladonna fails.

- *Hepar sulph*—mucus, pus in ear. For later stage of infection, when pus has developed behind the eardrum. Hates drafts, wants to cover ears or head. Chilly, oversensitive, sweats easily. Feels better with hot, damp weather.
- *Pulsatilla*—for a "ripe" (second or third stage) cold and ear infection. Copious, thick, yellow-green discharge. Changing symptoms. No thirst. Feels better in fresh, cold, open air; worse in warm, stuffy room. Feels worse in the evening.

When to consult a physician:

- If ear infections occur more than once or twice in a year.
- If ear infection and pain persist for more than four days.
- If ear infection is accompanied by a high fever (above 102°F).
- If the child has a stiff neck or arches the back.
- If the ear oozes pus or blood.
- If redness or swelling develops in the bony area behind the ear.

EYE INJURIES

The major causes of eye injuries include:

- sunburn
- foreign body
- bruising
- laceration

IMPORTANT: Eye injuries are very serious and require emergency care for all but the simplest of irritations.

Treatment for Sunburned Eyelids

Sunburn often occurs when someone falls asleep while sunbathing. This is one eye injury you may treat at home without concern about consulting a physician *unless the burn affects the eyeball.*

- Apply aloe vera or sliced cucumber to the eyelids. Be sure to keep aloe vera out of the eye itself.

Homeopathic remedies: 30c potency. Take three pellets 2–3 times per day until symptoms improve.

- *Hypericum*—for redness with extremely sensitive, burning pain; first-degree burn.
- *Ruta*—for burns to the eyeball. Administer while en route to the hospital.
- *Apis*—swollen lids. Profuse, hot tears. Photophobia (aversion to bright light), but can't bear covering eyes.

When to consult a physician:

- When the eyeball is affected.
- If the sunburned eyelid is blistered or looks charred.

Treatment for Foreign Bodies in the Eyes

These suggestions are for care en route to the hospital.

- Loosely patch both eyes, even if only one side is injured. Tight bandaging may cause the object to move deeper into the eye. Loosely bandaging both eyes reduces movement. (If only one eye is bandaged, both eyes will continue to move in response to what one eye sees.) You can use anything for a bandage, although a dry, sterile bandage is ideal. A clean T-shirt or other soft cloth will work in an emergency situation.
- If something is sticking out of the eye, cut a hole in the bottom of a paper cup and affix the lip of the cup to the facial surface (cheeks, forehead, etc.) surrounding the eye, with the object protruding through the hole in the cup. The cup will keep the object from moving and protect the eye from further damage.
- Never put ointment in the eye.
- For sand or grit, you may not need to go to the hospital if you are able to remove it by using one or more of the following suggestions:

1. Blink, up to 100 times. Blinking moves objects to the corners of the eye, where they are easy to remove.
2. Flood the eye with water.
3. Push up the lower lid, pull upper lid out and down (over the lower lid), then roll the eye. This will move the object to the center of the eye.
4. Touch the foreign body with a damp sterile cotton applicator (best), or a clean damp handkerchief or bandanna.
5. End with a Calendula wash—ten drops of *Calendula succus* in two tablespoons of water (best to use sterile water or saline solution).

Homeopathic remedies: 30c potency, three pellets 2–3 times per day until symptoms resolve.

- *Silica*—pushes out foreign objects

Herbs to soothe the eye after removing sand or grit: make a tea of euphrasia ("eyebright") by placing one tablespoon of dried herb (leaf) in a cup of boiling water. Steep for ten minutes, then strain through cheesecloth or other filtering material. Allow the tea to cool to room temperature, then flush the eye with tea using an eye cup (available at most pharmacies.). Make a new batch of tea each day.

Treatment for Bruises to the Eye

Administer the following treatments en route to the hospital.

General recommendations:

- Immediately apply washcloths wrung out in cold water, replacing as they are warmed by the eye; or apply tofu that has been in the refrigerator.
- After 24 hours, alternate hot and cold applications, five minutes with a warm washcloth, one minute with a cold washcloth. Repeat the cycle at least three times, always ending with a cold washcloth for one minute.

Homeopathic remedies: 30c potency. Take one dose of the remedy 2–3 times per day until symptoms improve.

- *Ruta*—is called the "Arnica of eye." For acute trauma or for slow healing of the eyeball. After serious injury, you can take *Ruta* every 20–60 minutes as required.
- *Hypericum*—for sharp, shooting nerve pain and numbness around eye.
- *Ledum*—black eye. Feels better with cold applications.
- *Aconite*—sudden heat. Feels anxious. Use during the first twenty-four hours after injury.

FEVER

Fever is a response to

- endogenous pyrogens (fever-causing chemicals produced in the body)
- bacteria
- exercise
- dehydration

The body produces endogenous pyrogens when bacteria or viruses overgrow in the body. These pyrogens signal the body to increase the core temperature. They also are responsible for many of the symptoms associated with a fever—achiness, fatigue, mental dullness. Again, these reactions can be seen as protective. Often the body needs rest more than anything else.

As mentioned earlier, the body knows that bacteria and viruses can survive only in a narrow temperature range. A fever creates an inhospitable environment for the pathogens. The inability to spike a fever in response to an infection is a sign of weakness and debility. Patients with serious diseases such as AIDS and cancer often do not have enough strength to generate a fever. Elderly people also may have serious infections without any signs of fever, also a sign of weakened vitality. Diagnosing infections in the elderly and in those with serious illnesses can be more difficult precisely because they cannot run a fever.

Elevated temperature in response to exercise is a normal reaction. In fact, this naturally generated "fever therapy" may help reduce infections during the cold and flu season. Fever due to dehydration, on the other hand, is never a healthy response. If you are working hard or exercising heavily outdoors in a hot climate, make sure that you are drinking plenty of fluids (at least 2–3 quarts per day).

Prolonged fever, especially in children, can produce brain damage. Serious diseases, however, may result from giving aspirin to children with high fevers. For example, Reye's syndrome, characterized by brain dysfunction (acute encephalopathy) and replacement of organs with fatty tissue (fatty degeneration of the viscera), can result from giving aspirin to feverish children suffering from viral infections. Obviously, not every child with a viral infection and fever who is given aspirin will manifest Reye's syndrome, but the risk of such side effects of aspirin is far greater than the risk associated with high fevers.

Parents often fear convulsions that may result from high fevers, but according to Dr. Alvin N. Eden, "a child who has a fever during a seizure does not have epilepsy. Furthermore, simple febrile seizures do not lead to mental retardation." In fact, reports pediatrician Uwe Stave, "Fever attacks can affect children in quite a positive way. Even though…physical strength is reduced, the child may disclose a wealth of new interests and skills. He may find new advanced ways to communicate, think, and handle situations, or display a refinement of his motor skills. In short, after a fever, the child reveals a spurt of development and maturation." (Both sources quoted in Rahima Baldwin, "Childhood Fevers," *Mothering*, Spring 1989, p. 36.)

Convulsions rarely occur in children when the fever runs at or below 102°F. The best approach is to work with the fever, keeping it in safe range, rather than giving aspirin or Tylenol to reduce it. Often anti-inflammatory drugs merely suppress a fever; afterward, the temperature can rebound even higher, especially with children. Choosing to use hydrotherapy or other therapeutics requires close monitoring of the child's temperature.

General recommendations:

- Drink plenty of fluids (two to four quarts per day).
- Rest. Stop your activities and go to bed ASAP.
- Stop eating. The proper translation of the old adage is "If you feed a cold, you will have to starve a fever." Digestion slows dramatically when the body spikes a fever. Food tends to ferment and putrefy, so the best treatment is to fast and drink plenty of fluids, allowing the body to use its energy to support the immune system rather than the digestive system.
- Encourage sweating (if your temperature is below 102°F) to break the fever and push out what the Chinese refer to as "external pernicious influences" (EPIs), which may include wind, dampness, heat, and cold. Simmer a tablespoon of fresh ginger in two cups of water for ten minutes. Draw a hot bath. Sip the ginger tea while relaxing in the bath. Once you begin to sweat, get out of the bath, towel dry, and get into bed. Wrap up in warm blankets and allow yourself to sweat. In the morning, take a shower to rinse off the sweat and excreted toxins.

  CAUTION: 1) Make sure that you are not exposed to drafts or chills during this treatment. Your pores are open and, therefore, more susceptible to drafts and chills. 2) Sweating therapy can further weaken someone who is debilitated, e.g., the elderly or those with long-term chronic illnesses. Also, children usually do not require such aggressive therapy.

- Continue resting for another twenty-four hours after your temperature returns to normal. The body needs time to recover fully. If people return to their busy schedules too quickly, they are often sick again with another round of cold or flu within six weeks.

Homeopathic remedies: 30c potency. Take three pellets 2–3 times per day until improvement is noted, then stop taking the remedy.

- *Aconite*—Hot, dry, cranky. Fever often develops after exposure to cold wind. Fearful, anxious.
- *Ferrum phos*—fever without other specific symptoms.
- *Belladonna*—glassy-eyed, dilated pupils; hot, red, dry face; sweaty body; possibly delirium. Sudden onset. No thirst. Specific for strep.

When a fever goes above 102°F:

- Place a cold washcloth on the forehead.
- Use a cold application on at least one-quarter of the body surface (see "Hydrotherapy" section of Chapter 2).
- Take a sponge bath in cool or tepid water, every 1–2 hours if necessary (especially with children).
- Soak the feet in a basin of cool or tepid water.
- Do not reduce a fever too quickly or too far. Remember, the optimal range for a fever is 99–102°F.
- Drink a glass of fluid (water is best) every hour.

When to consult a physician:

- If the fever persists more than three days.
- If the fever stays above 102°F, despite using the methods outlined above.
- If a child has a stiff neck, or is arching the back.

- If patient has other symptoms, such as burning urination, severe low-back pain, persistent sore throat (for longer than three days), or infected skin abrasions.

HEADACHE

Headaches may be caused by a variety of conditions. The suggestions below are meant for acute care, not to substitute for a thorough physical history and examination of those suffering with chronic headaches.

General recommendations:

- Progressive relaxation exercises. Many headaches are caused by muscle constriction and tension. Practice the following exercise during an acute headache and as a daily preventive measure:

Body Sweep

Sit or lie down in a comfortable position. Begin at the feet and slowly move through each body part—foot, ankle, calf, knee, thigh, etc.—noticing any areas of tension. When you sense a tight area, imagine the body becoming warm and heavy there. Continue moving toward the head until your entire body is warm and relaxed.

Once you have completed the "body sweep," imagine yourself relaxing in a favorite environment (by the ocean, in a shady forest, by a beautiful lake). Take a mini-vacation for at least five minutes in this favorite spot. When you are ready, return your attention to the room where you are sitting or lying, open your eyes, and take three deep breaths.

- Take a hot foot bath, or alternating hot and cold foot bath, to reduce congestion in the head area.
- Place a cold washcloth on the forehead. A cold application reduces congestion in the head. Combining a cold compress to the head with a hot foot bath will increase the effect of the treatment.

- Rub a drop of essential oil of lavender into each temple.
- Drink lots of water, a minimum of two to three quarts per day. Some headaches are caused by simple dehydration.
- Increase fiber (whole grains, fruits, and vegetables) in the diet. Constipation may cause reabsorption of toxins, leading to "sick headaches." Be sure to increase water consumption so that increased fiber does not bind the stools.
- Eliminate coffee, cola, and black tea from the diet. These are common contributors to headaches. Migraines are the exception: caffeine causes blood-vessel constriction, which reduces early migraine symptoms. (Most migraines are caused by excessive dilation of blood vessels; common headaches are caused by blood-vessel constriction.)
- Tobacco causes blood-vessel constriction. Reduce or eliminate cigarette smoking, tobacco chewing, etc.
- Acupressure stimulation of the following points:
  1. Large Intestine 4: the web between the thumb and first finger.
  2. Liver 3: the web between the first and second toe.
  3. *Yin tang*: just above the bridge of the nose.
  4. *Tai yang*: the temple area on either side of the forehead.
  5. Stomach 36: just below the knee on the lateral (outer) side, one finger breadth away from the shin bone.
- Keep the extremities (arms and legs) warm.
- Take a brisk walk in the fresh air, being sure to keep the extremities warm (mittens, hat, scarf, and boots in winter months).
- Drink red clover or catnip tea at the first sign of a headache.

Homeopathic remedies: 30c potency

- *Belladonna*—Intense, throbbing pain. Extreme sensitivity to noise, light, touch, strong smells. Pain comes on suddenly, usually in the frontal area. Pain may extend to the back of the head. Feels worse after jarring. Face may be red and hot, extremities cold. Pupils may be dilated.

- *Bryonia*—worse with any motion, even slight movement of the head or eyes. Better with firm pressure to the painful area. Steady, aching pain may be concentrated over the left eye or over the forehead area. Irritable, wants to be left alone. Improves with warmth.
- *Nux vomica*—for headaches following excesses in eating or drinking; hangovers. Generally sick feeling, with possible digestive upset. Aversion to light and sound. Avoids company. Irritable.
- *Gelsemium*—Heavy head, as if full of molasses. Dull headache. Sensation of having a band around the head. Joints are achy, heavy. Wants to be alone.

INDIGESTION

Indigestion usually results from eating too much food, or eating the wrong kinds of food for our particular bodies. The best treatment is preventive—eat fresh, well-cooked foods prepared and eaten in a relaxed environment. Avoid arguments while eating. Chew each bite well (some say at least fifty times). Some days, I'm lucky if I chew each bite ten times! Eat while sitting down, preferably in a chair, and not while hurtling along the freeway in your car. Remember that the digestive system works best when we are relaxed, which is when the parasympathetic nervous system is most active (see the section on "Nutrition" in Chapter 2).

- Avoid eating when you are rushed or emotionally upset. The body shunts energy and circulation away from the digestive tract during stressful periods, whether the stress is physical, mental, or emotional.
- Avoid eating excessive amounts of cold or raw food. From a Chinese medical perspective, the stomach functions best when it is warm (but not overheated). Steamed and baked foods are easiest to digest. Raw foods, as well as cold or

frozen foods, tend to be very cooling and therefore difficult to digest. In general, the body tolerates a modest
amount of raw food better in the warm summer months
than during the winter.

- Avoid highly spiced, fried, or greasy foods, which may over-
heat the digestive system and cause irritation.
- Choose water and herb teas for beverages. Avoid coffee,
black tea, and alcohol, all of which are heating and irritating to the digestive tract.

Botanical therapy:

- *Peppermint oil*—one drop in a cup of hot water. Essential
oils are very strong, so one drop really is enough.
- *Ginger tea*—grate one or two tablespoons of fresh ginger
into two cups of water. Bring to a boil and simmer for ten
minutes. Sip the warm tea as needed. Ginger is warming,
which helps stimulate digestion.
- *Chamomile and/or mint tea*—add one tablespoon of dried
herb to one cup of boiling water. Allow to steep for ten
minutes, then drink.
- *"Pill Curing"*—a Chinese patent formula. Take one vial of
the pellets every 3–4 hours as needed.

Homeopathic remedies: 30c potency

- *Nux vomica*—classic for overeating and overdrinking. The
patient tends to overwork and keep a demanding schedule,
which irritates his already weak digestive system. Tendency
to constipation.
- *Arsenicum*—burning pain in the stomach, with desire to
drink small sips of water, although water may cause vomiting. Food poisoning with both diarrhea and vomiting.

When to consult a physician:

- If indigestion becomes a regular occurrence (more than
once or twice per week).
- If you notice changes in the bowel movements.

- Black, tarry stools (may be an indication of stomach or duodenal ulcer).
- Excessive gas and bloating (may be an indication of parasite infection). This does not include gas caused by eating too many or poorly cooked beans!
- Regular or severe episodes of heartburn.
- If symptoms of indigestion, bloating, and burping consistently follow ingestion of fatty, greasy, or rich foods (may be a symptom of gall bladder irritation).

INSECT AND OTHER BITES

In general, clean the wound with soap and water.

Botanical therapy:

- *Calendula succus* (plant juice, preserved with a small amount of alcohol)—encourages wound healing and prevents infection. Apply after washing the bite.
- *Comfrey or mullein compresses*—also encourage healing. Comfrey contains allantoin, a plant constituent that increases cell division and thereby speeds wound healing. Mullein has soothing properties to ease the stinging and itching associated with insect bites. Make a compress by crushing the leaves or putting fresh leaves in the blender with a small amount of water. Spread the crushed leaves on muslin or cheesecloth and apply to the affected area.
- *Fresh potato*—cut in slices and apply to affected areas to draw out inflammation and swelling.
- *Bentonite clay*—reconstituted to a paste and applied to the area, this will draw out inflammation and swelling and reduce pain.

Homeopathic remedies: 30c potency

- *Ledum*—specific for bites and puncture wounds of all kinds, especially those that are cold and pale blue in color. Ledum is especially helpful for "dirty" bites, or animals bites that are susceptible to infection.

- *Cantharis*—bites with intense itching, small red bumps, vesicles.
- *Tarantula*—for spider bites.
- *Apis*—for bee stings, or any kind of sting that causes intense, painful swelling and stinging.
- *Hypericum*—for shooting pain.
- *Lachesis*—for snake bite.

When to consult a physician:
- If the insect bite becomes infected.
- If you have an allergic reaction to the insect sting, e.g., excessive swelling in the local area or difficulty breathing.
- If you suspect you may have been bitten by a poisonous insect.

MENSTRUAL CRAMPING

From the perspective of Chinese medicine, stagnation leads to pain. Stagnation may be caused by cold or, paradoxically, by a decrease in the cooling, nourishing *yin* fluids of the body. A deficiency of blood, a yin substance, causes irritation, cramping, and scanty blood flow. The deficiency is a qualitative decrease in blood, not a quantitative deficiency that would show up on a blood test.

Cold also causes constriction. Generally, cramping worsens with cold, whether the source of the cold is internal or external.

- Avoid cold foods and drinks the week before menses begins. Cold causes constriction and exacerbates cramping, whether the source of the cold is internal (food and drink) or external (cold drafts, swimming in cold water, etc.).
- Exercise is a good preventive, increasing circulation and decreasing stagnation.
- Clear your schedule as much as possible the day before you begin bleeding. If possible, have a completely quiet, unscheduled day when you begin bleeding.

Botanical therapy:

- *Yarrow*—acts as a diuretic for bloating associated with premenstrual syndrome (PMS).
- *Wild yam*—to reduce cramping and balance hormones.
- *Valerian officinalis*—to reduce cramping and relax smooth muscles. (The uterus is smooth muscle tissue.)
- *Red raspberry leaf*—uterine tonic.

Combine equal parts of the above. Drink three to four cups of tea per day, or take two dropperfuls every 1–2 hours during acute, severe cramping.

Nutritional therapy:

- Increase fiber in the diet. Slow, sluggish bowels encourage the re-uptake of hormones the body is trying to excrete through the intestines. High hormonal levels may exacerbate menstrual cramping, as well as PMS symptoms.
- Drink at least two quarts of water per day to increase elimination from the body.
- Eat magnesium-rich foods. Magnesium encourages muscle relaxation.
- Take 50–100 mg of vitamin B_6 per day for at least two months.
- Exercise aerobically at least twenty minutes, 3–4 times per week. Exercise increases circulation in the reproductive organs and decreases stress levels, both of which can decrease menstrual cramping.

Homeopathic remedies: 30c potency

- *Belladonna*—heavy sensation in abdomen. Menses bright red, profuse. Restless. Head sensitive to drafts. Feels worse after jarring or even when touched.
- *Borax*—fears downward motion. Membrane and tissue pass with menses. Early, profuse bleeding, with colic and nausea. Application of pressure eases discomfort. Feels better during cold weather.

- *Bryonia*—"vicarious menses," i.e., nosebleed rather than menstrual flow. Inter-menses pains with pelvic and abdominal soreness. Avoids the least motion. Thirsty for large amounts of water.
- *Calc phos*—violent backache. Chilly. Menses is early, excessive, bright red; occurs every two weeks.
- *Chamomilla*—dark, clotted blood with labor-like pains. Irritable, cross, quarrelsome. Thirsty. Feels worse at night, when angry, or after drinking coffee.
- *Colocynthis*—Patient bends over double; pain "bores into" ovary. Pain eases with pressure. Restless. Waves of violent, gripping pain.
- *Pulsatilla*—sensation of band around throat just before menses. Clotted, intermittent, changeable menses.

When to consult a physician:

- If severe menstrual cramping occurs more than twice in a year.
- If menstrual cramping worsens over time (possible indication that endometriosis may be developing).
- If the cramps are severe enough to stop your daily activities.

MOTION SICKNESS

General recommendations:

- Relaxation exercises, before and during travel. Move through the body from head to foot, noting and releasing any areas of muscle tension. Take up to ten deep breaths and allow your body to grow heavy and relaxed.
- Drink ginger tea. Grate one or two tablespoons of fresh ginger into a saucepan with two cups of water. Bring to a boil, then simmer for ten minutes. Drink one-half cup of ginger tea every half hour, or as needed for stomach upset.
- Mint and chamomile teas also soothe the stomach. Steep one tablespoon dried herb in a cup of boiling water for ten minutes. Drink as needed.

Homeopathic remedies: 30c potency. Take the remedy one hour before travel, then every 15–30 minutes as needed once travel begins.

- *Borax*—for motion sickness during air travel. Symptoms worsen with downward motion.
- *Rhus tox*—nausea and vomiting with complete loss of appetite. Giddiness on attempting to rise. Severe frontal headache. Unquenchable thirst.
- *Cocculus*—for car sickness. Also for morning sickness in pregnancy. Person cannot stand the sight or smell of food. Hollow, empty feeling.

When to consult a physician:

- If the above remedies do not alleviate motion sickness.
- If you have difficulties with balance that are exacerbated by travel. You may have an inner-ear problem that needs further treatment.

PHYSICAL TRAUMA

Most trauma is caused by stretching tissues beyond their capacity. Overstretching connective tissues (muscle, blood vessels, tendons, bones) leads to tissue damage, pain, and swelling. Swelling may serve as a natural splint, to protect and immobilize the traumatized area. Unfortunately, swelling may also lead to a dangerous decrease in circulation.

The treatments listed below apply to most physical injuries. Please see other sections of this chapter for information on specific conditions (bruising, burns, etc.).

- Give homeopathic *Arnica* as soon as possible after the injury. *Arnica* is specific for trauma, bruising, head injury, and soft-tissue injury, and can also slow bleeding and treat shock. Often someone needing *Arnica* will deny that she is injured. Imagine a construction worker falling two stories, landing hard, getting up, and saying she is fine—she needs *Arnica*!

- Continue giving *Arnica* as needed for 3–4 days. You may repeat the remedy as often as every thirty minutes immediately after the injury. Remember, homeopathic remedies act according to the frequency of dosage, not the amount.
- For the first twenty-four hours, use cold applications to the affected area. There is some controversy here: one school of thought says cold applications are best because they reduce circulation, and therefore swelling, in the local area; another school of thought argues that cold applications cause "stagnation" (as defined in Chinese medicine) by slowing the circulation. A compromise approach involves alternating hot and cold applications to increase circulation and decrease stagnation.
- After twenty-four hours, use alternating hot and cold applications—five minutes of hot, followed by one minute of cold. Continue for at least three cycles of alternating hot and cold applications. Always end with a cold application.

Other Homeopathic remedies: 30c potency

- *Ledum*—bruised area that is cold and blue. Follows *Arnica* well, after three or four days.
- *Ruta*—injury to periosteal tissue (surface of the bone). Area is red; condition worsens with motion. Also for injuries to ligaments.
- *Rhus tox*—sore, painful joints that improve with warmth and motion (painful when first moved, better with continued movement).
- *Hypericum*—for injury to areas dense with nerve tissue (eyes, hands, genitals). Sharp, nerve-like pain.

Botanical remedies:

- *Arnica oil*—apply to the affected area every 3–4 hours. Because Arnica is a counter-irritant (increasing circulation in an area by causing mild irritation) it should not be used on broken skin.

CAUTION: for external use only. Do not take Arnica internally. Use on unbroken skin only.

- *Hypericum oil*—causes blood-vessel dilation; warming to injured area, soothing to nerves. CAUTION: for external use only.

- *Symphytum (comfrey) oil or lotion*—stimulates cell production and tissue healing. Apply externally, or take as tea internally. Comfrey tea is especially healing for bone breaks. CAUTION: for skin injuries (cuts and abrasions), apply comfrey only after scab formation. Applying comfrey to a deep, open wound can cause the wound to close too quickly, trapping anaerobic bacteria in the wound and possibly causing a serious infection.

- Any plant with chlorophyll will stimulate healing. Plantain is exceptionally soothing to the skin. Crush the leaves and apply to cuts and abrasions, especially if you are outdoors and have no other first-aid supplies with you. Plantain is called "nature's Band-Aid."

Acupressure: Deeply massage points on the limb opposite the injured area. Massaging points on the left wrist will decrease pain and increase circulation to a sprained right wrist.

When to consult a physician:

- If the patient shows signs of shock (see the section on "Shock," below).
- If the injury involves blood loss (more than minor oozing from a cut).
- If you cannot voluntarily move the injured area.
- If you can see bone protruding through the skin.
- If you begin to see red streaks developing above an injury, moving up the arm or leg—a sign of internal infection.
- If pain and swelling persist for more than 3–4 days after injury.

POISON IVY AND POISON OAK

General recommendations:

- Learn to identify these plants and keep a respectful distance away from them.
- Wash with soap and water. The rash and irritation associated with poison oak and ivy are caused by an oil in the plant's leaves and stems. Washing with soap, which emulsifies and removes oils, decreases and sometimes completely removes the irritant.
- Remove the irritant with drawing agents. Moisten bentonite clay with enough water to form a smooth paste. Add one or two drops of peppermint oil. The clay will absorb oils and oozing discharge from poison ivy rashes. A very small amount of peppermint oil will decrease itching. If you do not have clay, apply a fresh slice of potato to the area. (Potato also acts as a drawing agent.)
- Avoid touching or brushing the affected area. You may spread the irritant oil accidentally by scratching the rash, then touching another body part. This is usually how poison ivy spreads to the eyes and face. If you tend to scratch in your sleep, wear cotton gloves. Wash your hands often during the day.

Homeopathic remedies: 30c potency

- *Rhus tox*—for itchy, red vesicles. The area feels better with hot-water applications and motion.
- *Rhus lobatum*—made from poison oak, which is more common on the West Coast. Some people respond better to this remedy than to *Rhus tox*, which is made from poison ivy.
- If you are extremely sensitive to poison ivy or oak and must work in or near it (e.g., clearing poison ivy in your yard), take one 30c dose of *Rhus tox* before beginning work. This prophylactic dose can reduce and sometimes prevent a rash.

When to consult a physician:
- If the rash continues to spread despite treatment.
- If the rash persists for more than seven days.
- If the area becomes infected.

SHOCK

When someone goes into shock, the body suspends all but the most vital functions. If shock goes untreated, even those vital functions may shut down. Symptoms of shock include:
- confusion
- very slow or very fast pulse
- very slow or very fast breathing
- trembling or weakness of the arms and legs
- cool, moist skin
- enlarged pupils
- pale or bluish fingernails, lips, skin

Treatments for shock:

Call 911. Most shock is caused by major trauma and requires immediate medical attention. The following suggestions are meant to support the patient until emergency medical care arrives.
- Keep the patient lying down.
- Address the cause of the shock: remove any live electrical source (if you can do so without endangering yourself), stanch bleeding, remove causes of severe pain, use first-aid procedures to restore breathing.
- Keep the patient warm. Cover him or her with a blanket, and elevate the feet.
- Give "Rescue Remedy," a blend of Bach flowers available at most health-food stores. Give three or four drops under the tongue every fifteen minutes, or as necessary once recovery begins.

Homeopathic remedies: 30c potency. Give every 15–30 minutes until improvement is noted.

- *Aconite*—fear, fright, anxiety. Sudden, violent onset. Numbness. Vomiting from fear. Face is deathly pale when patient sits up. Fear of death.
- *Carbo veg*—icy coldness. Stagnant blood. "Air hunger" (can't catch breath). Wants windows open; wants to be fanned; wants cold drinks during chills.
- *Gelsemium*—dull, droopy, drowsy, dazed. Dilated pupils. No thirst. Heat stroke. Heavy, drooping eyelids.
- *Arnica*—especially after head injury. Denies need for help ("I'm fine. Just leave me alone.").

When to consult a physician:

- Always consult a physician for illnesses and injuries involving shock.
- If the patient has minor injuries (e.g., a scraped leg or arm) and does not respond to the above treatment within 10–15 minutes.

SUNBURN

Fair-skinned people always have been susceptible to sunburn. Now, with the increasing emissions of hydrocarbons and fluorocarbons and subsequent destruction of the ozone layer, even dark-skinned people are at risk. The long-term effects of excessive sun exposure include skin cancer. One severe sunburn during a lifetime can increase the risk of multiple myeloma, i.e., bone cancer. The best treatment is preventive:

- Stay out of the sun during the middle of the day (11 a.m.– 3 p.m.), when the sun's rays are strongest.
- Wear hats that screen the face, especially the nose. Wear light clothing that covers the arms and legs.

- Apply sunscreen to areas of the skin that are not covered by clothing. Sunscreen increases the number of minutes the skin can withstand burning rays by the factor noted on the product. For example, a fair-skinned person without protection might normally stay in the sun for ten minutes before noticing signs of burning. If that person uses a "15" sunscreen, he or she could stay in the sun for 10 x 15 minutes, or 150 minutes (i.e., two-and-a-half hours). Reapplying the sunscreen after 150 minutes will not increase the length of protection. Washing off the sunscreen will reduce the effective time.

If you are unable to avoid overexposure, use the following treatments:

- Apply cool water as soon as possible. Take frequent cool showers (e.g., two minutes in the shower, every one or two hours). Pat dry; do not rub the skin. If the burn is localized, apply cold wet washcloths, changing the cloth as it warms.
- Apply aloe vera gel every 3–4 hours.
- Avoid applications of oil-based products or butter. Oils and fats increase the burn, just as throwing grease on a fire will feed the flames.
- Drink plenty of fluids. Often the body becomes dehydrated, especially if the burn covers a large area of the body.

Homeopathic remedies: 30c potency

- *Hypericum*—for first-degree sunburn (no blistering).
- *Cantharis*—especially if blistering is present (second-degree burn)

When to consult a physician:

- If a second-degree burn (i.e., with blistering) covers more than 10 percent of the skin surface.
- If the patient shows signs of:
  a. heat stroke—collapse in the heat with hot, dry skin. Other symptoms include a rapid, strong pulse and high body

temperature (105°F or higher). Heat stroke is a very serious condition requiring immediate medical attention.

b. heat exhaustion—collapse in the heat with moist, clammy skin. Other symptoms include profuse perspiration, weakness, nausea, dizziness, headaches, and possibly cramps. Heat exhaustion is a serious condition, although not as life-threatening as heat stroke.

TEETHING

Many symptoms may accompany the eruption of teeth in an infant, including colds, ear infections, and diarrhea. The following suggestions are meant specifically for the gum and mouth symptoms.

- Soak a clean cloth in chamomile tea, wring out, and place in the freezer. Give to baby to chew on when he or she shows signs of discomfort.
- Water-filled plastic "teething rings" can soothe inflamed gums.
- If you are breast feeding, drink chamomile and oatstraw tea (equal parts). The herbs will pass into the breast milk.

Homeopathic remedies: 30c potency

- *Calc carb*—late dentition (teeth slow to emerge). Fontanelles slow to close. Ear infections sometimes accompany teething.
- *Chamomilla*—a classic remedy for teething, especially for inconsolable children, or children who are extremely irritable and demand to be carried, yet arch their back away from whomever is carrying them. One cheek is red, the other pale. Grass-green, runny stools may accompany teething.
- *Ignatia*—child is distressed, but not as irritable as in previous case. The baby sobs, sighs, and cries. The whole body—or single body parts—may tremble.

Chapter Four
How To Choose a Naturopathic Physician

Choosing a physician is like choosing a car—you need someone you can trust who will take you where you need to go. As with any human relationship, "chemistry" is part of the equation. Your dream physician may be like the flashy sports car, or the car with the best gas mileage, or the one with the sensible upholstery.

In all states in which naturopathic physicians are licensed, they function as primary-care physicians, meaning they are qualified to diagnose and treat disease. The naturopathic doctor (N.D.) functions as a family doctor, the equivalent to conventional medicine's general practitioner (G.P.). A naturopathic physician employs physical exams, patient health histories, and lab tests to arrive at diagnoses, just like any other physician. An N.D. varies from conventional medical practice only in the treatments that he or she prescribes to address illness. In some states, naturopathic physicians may prescribe pharmaceutical drugs.

In states without a naturopathic licensing board, anyone may call him or herself a "naturopathic doctor," or use the initials "N.D." after his or her name, because the term is not legally defined or regulated by the state. Before making an appointment with an N.D., ask where he or she went to school. In North America, there are three accredited four-year schools of naturopathic medicine. Physicians who have graduated from one of these schools have completed a rigorous medical training, equivalent to that offered at conventional medical schools, with the addition of natural therapeutic modalities absent from most medical school curricula (see Appendix for comparison chart). Check with the schools listed below or with the American Association of Naturopathic Physicians (AANP) to find a trained naturopathic physician in an unlicensed state.

In licensed states, naturopathic physicians must pass a national board exam (three days of written exams) before they are licensed. Most naturopathic physicians who have graduated from an accredited school pass national board exams and retain a license in a licensed state, even if they are practicing in a state that does not recognize naturopathic physicians.

States presently licensing naturopathic physicians include: Alaska, Arizona, Connecticut, Florida, Hawaii, Maine, Montana, New Hampshire, Oregon, Utah, and Washington. The following Canadian provinces license naturopathic physicians: Alberta, British Columbia, Manitoba, Ontario, Quebec, and Saskatchewan.

Keep in mind that each licensed naturopathic physician is likely to emphasize particular therapeutic approaches in his or her practice. Always ask what therapeutic methods a particular practitioner uses (e.g., nutrition, homeopathy, botanical medicine, physical medicine, hydrotherapy, etc.). I know of one patient who went to a naturopathic physician for several months, always expecting that the physician eventually would prescribe a homeopathic remedy. Finally, this extremely patient patient asked the physician when he was going to prescribe a remedy. "Oh," said the physician, arching his eyebrow in surprise, "I don't work with homeopathic remedies. I suggest you contact Dr. So-and-so!"

General guidelines for choosing a physician (of any kind):

- The physician listens well and encourages questions.
- The physician asks what *you* think is happening with your health.
- The physician takes time to explain things.
- The treatment plan includes lifestyle changes, not just pills.
- The physician outlines options and helps you make educated health-care choices.
- The physician educates patients during an office visit and, ideally, also offers lectures and trainings for patients who desire more information.
- The physician conducts physical exams and orders appropriate lab tests. This does not apply to naturopathic physicians in unlicensed states, where N.D.s must refer patients to other physicians for lab testing. In licensed states, naturopathic physicians can order lab tests, draw blood, etc.

Accredited North American naturopathic medical schools:

Bastyr University
14500 Juanita Drive NE
Bothell, WA 98011
(206) 823-1300

National College of Naturopathic Medicine
Ross Island Center
049 S.W. Porter
Portland, OR 97201
(503) 225-4860

Ontario College of Naturopathic Medicine
60 Berl Avenue
Toronto, Ontario M8Y3C7
Canada
(416) 251-5261

Currently undergoing accreditation:
> Southwest College of Naturopathic Medicine and
>   Health Sciences
> 2140 East Broadway Road
> Tempe, AZ 85282
> (602) 990-7424

American Association of Naturopathic Physicians (AANP)
referral line: (206) 323-7610

APPENDIX
Naturopathic and
Major Medical Schools

Comparative Curricula of Classroom and Clinical Hours

Naturopathic Schools:	National College of Naturopathic Medicine	Bastyr College (Naturopathic)
Basic and Clinical Sciences including Anatomy, Cell Biology, Physiology, Pathology, Neurosciences Clinical/Physical Diagnosis, Histology, Genetics, Biochemistry, Pharmacology, Biostatistics, Epidemiology, Public Health, History, Philosophy, Ethics, Research, and other coursework.	2070	1891
Clerkships and Allopathic Therapeutics including lecture and clinical instruction in Dermatology, Family Medicine, Psychiatry, Medicine, Radiology, Pediatrics, Obstetrics, Gynecology, Neurology, Minor Surgery, Ophthalmology, and clinical electives.	1974	1959
Naturopathic Therapeutics including Botanical Medicine, Homeopathy, Oriental Medicine, Hydrotherapy, Naturopathic Manipulative Therapy.	492	335
Therapeutic Nutrition	144	138
Counseling	144	158
TOTALS	4824	4481

Sources: 1988 *Curriculum Directory* of the Association of American Medical Colleges. 1988 catalogues of National College of Naturopathic Medicine and Bastyr College.

Major Medical Schools:	John Hopkins	Mayo	Yale	Stanford
Basic and Clinical Sciences including Anatomy, Cell Biology, Physiology, Pathology, Neurosciences Clinical/Physical Diagnosis, Histology, Genetics, Biochemistry, Pharmacology, Biostatistics, Epidemiology, Public Health, History, Philosophy, Ethics, Research, and other coursework.	1794	1640	1457	1401
Clerkships and Allopathic Therapeutics including lecture and clinical instruction in Dermatology, Family Medicine, Psychiatry, Medicine, Radiology, Pediatrics, Obstetrics, Gynecology, Neurology, Minor Surgery, Ophthalmology, and clinical electives.	3260	3080	2040 (+ thesis)	3840
Naturopathic Therapeutics including Botanical Medicine, Homeopathy, Oriental Medicine, Hydrotherapy, Naturopathic Manipulative Therapy.	0	0	0	0
Therapeutic Nutrition	17	elective	elective	elective
Counseling	0	0 (included under psychiatry above)	0	0
TOTALS	5071	4720	3497 (+ thesis)	5241

For Information or Referrals: American Association of Naturopathic Physicians, P.O. Box 20386, Seattle, WA 98102, (206) 323-7610

BIBLIOGRAPHY

This bibliography includes good introductory books to continue your exploration of naturopathic medicine. The list is by no means complete, but rather the beginning of a good home reference library for using natural therapeutics. The starred (*) references are for more advanced studies.

General

Murray, Michael, N.D. *Encyclopedia of Natural Medicine*. Rocklin, CA: Prima, 1991.

Mind, Emotions, Spirit

Borysenko, Joan. *Minding the Body, Mending the Mind*. New York: Bantam, 1988.

Cousins, Norman. *The Biology of Hope*. New York: Dutton, 1989.

Hanh, Thich Nhat. *The Blooming of a Lotus*. Boston: Beacon Press, 1993.

Myss, Caroline. *The Creation of Health*. Walpole, NH: Stillpoint, 1988.

Orioli, Esther et al. *Stress Map*. New York: Newmarket Press, 1991.

Siegel, Bernie, M.D. *Love, Medicine, and Miracles*. New York: Harper & Row, 1986.

Exercise

Anderson, Bob. *Stretching*. Bolinas, CA: Shelter Publications, 1980.

Bailey, Covert. *The New Fit or Fat*. Boston: Houghton Mifflin, 1991.

Cooper, Kenneth, M.D. *The New Aerobics*. New York: Bantam Books, 1978.

Iyengar, D.K.S. *Light on Yoga*. New York: Schocken Books, 1976.

The Sivananda Yoga Center. *The Book of Yoga*. London: Ebury Press, 1983.

Nutrition

Erasmus, Udo. *Fats and Oils*. Blaine, WA: Alive Books, 1986.

Murray, Michael, N.D. *The Healing Power of Foods*. Rocklin, CA: Prima Publishing, 1993.

Robbins, John. *Diet for a New America*. Walpole, NH: Stillpoint, 1987.

Hydrotherapy

Thrash, Agatha, and Thrash, Calvin. *Home Remedies*. Yuchi Pines, AL: Yuchi Pines Institute Health Education Department, 1981.

*Boyle, Wade. *Lectures in Naturopathic Hydrotherapy*. East Palestine, OH: Buckeye Naturopathic Press.

Botanical Medicine

Hoffmann, David. *The Holistic Herbal*. Longmead, England: Element Books, 1988.

Tierra, Michael. *The Way of Herbs*. New York: Pocket Books, 1983.

Tierra, Michael. *Planetary Herbology*. Santa Fe, NM: Lotus Press, 1988.

*Mrs. M. Grieve. *A Modern Herbal*. New York: Penguin, 1984 (first published 1931).

Homeopathic Medicine

Cummings, Stephen. *Everybody's Guide to Homeopathic Medicines.* Los Angeles: Tarcher, 1984.

Panos, Maesimund, M.D. *Homeopathic Medicine at Home.* Los Angeles: Tarcher, 1980.

*Tyler, Margaret Lucy. *Pointers to the Common Remedies.* Fremont, CA: Jain, 1993.

Physical Therapies

Downing, George. *The Massage Book.* New York: Random House, 1972.

Prudden, Bonnie. *Pain Erasure.* New York: Ballantine Books, 1980.

Tappan, Frances. *Healing Massage Techniques, Second Edition.* Norwalk, CT: Appleton & Lang, 1988.

Chinese Medicine

Haas, Elson. *Staying Healthy with the Seasons.* Berkeley, CA: Celestial Arts, 1981.

Kaptchuk, Ted. *The Web That Has No Weaver.* New York: Congdon & Weed, 1983.

*Maciocia, Giovanni. *The Foundations of Chinese Medicine.* New York: Churchill Livingstone, 1989.

Ayurvedic Medicine

Lad, Vasant, Dr. *Ayurveda: The Science of Self-Healing.* Santa Fe, NM: Lotus Press, 1984.

Chopra, Deepak, M.D. *Perfect Health.* New York: Harmony Books, 1991.

Other pocket guides from The Crossing Press

Pocket Guide to Ayurvedic Healing
By Candis Cantin Packard
$6.95 • Paper • ISBN 0-89594-764-1

Pocket Guide to Good Food
By Margaret M. Wittenberg
$6.95 • Paper • ISBN 0-89594-747-1

Pocket Herbal Reference Guide
By Debra Nuzzi
$6.95 • Paper • ISBN 0-89594-568-1

Pocket Guide to Aromatherapy
By Kathi Keville
$6.95 • Paper • ISBN 0-89594-815-X

Pocket Guide to Astrology
By Alan Oken
$6.95 • Paper • ISBN 0-89594-820-6

Pocket Guide to Numerology
By Alan Oken
$6.95 • Paper • ISBN 0-89594-826-5

Pocket Guide to the Tarot
By Alan Oken
$6.95 • Paper • 0-89594-822-2

Please look for these books at your local bookstore or order from
The Crossing Press, P.O. Box 1048, Freedom, CA 95019.
Add $2.50 for the first book and 50¢ for each additional book.
Or call toll-free 800-777-1048 with your credit card order.